Rakesh Dubey

Fundamental of Transosseous Fixation of Intercondylar Fracture Humerus

AF141267

Rakesh Dubey

Fundamental of Transosseous Fixation of Intercondylar Fracture Humerus

LAP LAMBERT Academic Publishing

Impressum / Imprint

Bibliografische Information der Deutschen Nationalbibliothek: Die Deutsche Nationalbibliothek verzeichnet diese Publikation in der Deutschen Nationalbibliografie; detaillierte bibliografische Daten sind im Internet über http://dnb.d-nb.de abrufbar.

Alle in diesem Buch genannten Marken und Produktnamen unterliegen warenzeichen-, marken- oder patentrechtlichem Schutz bzw. sind Warenzeichen oder eingetragene Warenzeichen der jeweiligen Inhaber. Die Wiedergabe von Marken, Produktnamen, Gebrauchsnamen, Handelsnamen, Warenbezeichnungen u.s.w. in diesem Werk berechtigt auch ohne besondere Kennzeichnung nicht zu der Annahme, dass solche Namen im Sinne der Warenzeichen- und Markenschutzgesetzgebung als frei zu betrachten wären und daher von jedermann benutzt werden dürften.

Bibliographic information published by the Deutsche Nationalbibliothek: The Deutsche Nationalbibliothek lists this publication in the Deutsche Nationalbibliografie; detailed bibliographic data are available in the Internet at http://dnb.d-nb.de.

Any brand names and product names mentioned in this book are subject to trademark, brand or patent protection and are trademarks or registered trademarks of their respective holders. The use of brand names, product names, common names, trade names, product descriptions etc. even without a particular marking in this work is in no way to be construed to mean that such names may be regarded as unrestricted in respect of trademark and brand protection legislation and could thus be used by anyone.

Coverbild / Cover image: www.ingimage.com

Verlag / Publisher:
LAP LAMBERT Academic Publishing
ist ein Imprint der / is a trademark of
OmniScriptum GmbH & Co. KG
Heinrich-Böcking-Str. 6-8, 66121 Saarbrücken, Deutschland / Germany
Email: info@lap-publishing.com

Herstellung: siehe letzte Seite /
Printed at: see last page
ISBN: 978-3-659-71536-5

Fundamentals of Transosseous Fixation of Intercondylar Fractures of Humerus

Author

Dr Rakesh R. Dubey,

MS (Ortho), DNB (Ortho)

Honorary Orthopaedic Surgeon - Department of Orthopaedics,
Shri Harilal Bhagwati Municipal General Hospital

Director - Dhanvantri Fracture, Maternity and General Hospital
Borivali (W), Mumbai 400092 - INDIA

PREFACE

"Transosseous Technique" is the first manuscript of this kind that aims to apprise its readers, the value of fixation around the elbow. Orthopaedic is rapidly evolving and changing medical science which is reaching out to new frontiers every day. The continuous innovations in instrumentation and advances suggest that we are just at the tip of the iceberg. The present work would help surgeons to reach their goal of treating the patient to the fullest. The work is based on the sound principles of physics. It would help to aim surgeons to achieve the most stable fixations around elbow. This book gives clear picture of the technique in simple sound language. This technique is simple to master and it doesn't require use of the expensive implants for fixation, yet giving better fixation results than other expensive implants. This technique can be called *friendly technique* as other fixation techniques can be simultaneously used along with this fixation technique.

For better understanding we have included the anatomical images, the CT scan images, radiological images and operative photographs. The book begins with the introductory session about the principles of the technique followed by, a brief anatomy of the elbow joint, clinical evaluation of injury, detailed operative technique and finally concluding with detailed discussion about the fixation technique. This fixation technique could open a plethora of research opportunities in dealing with the fracture fixations in other region also.

A new technique and a new text book might contain errors and weakness—we welcome your corrections and suggestions for future editions.

The only purpose to publish this novel technique in form of a book is to help my colleagues to utilize this technique for the betterment of mankind.

I hope you enjoy reading this book as much as I have enjoyed writing it.

Dr. Rakesh Dubey

M.S (Ortho), DNB (Ortho)

ACKNOWLEDGEMENTS

I take this opportunity to express my sincere and heartfelt gratitude for the love and support by my wife Dr Shweta Dubey and my kids Atharva and Shrishti for the constant inspiration and support. I am extremely thankful for their affection, confidence in me and for their invaluable suggestions in showing me the correct direction. I am also very thankful to them for helping me out in hard situations and compelling me to publish this work.

I express my gratitude to all my colleagues and residents for the support. Last but not the least I express my thanks to all my patients to whom I have served. I apologise from the depth of my heart if I hurt anyone knowingly or unknowingly. Especially I want to thank my residents Dr. Jainil Parmar and Dr. Sandeep Sonawane for their contribution.

I sincerely want to dedicate this work to my parents Dr Ramakant Dubey and late. Smt. Phulvatidevi Dubey, without their blessings this work would not have been possible.

This task would not have been completed without the grace of almighty, the most beneficent and most merciful, the best healer.

CONTENT

INTRODUCTION

Low metaphyseal and intraarticular fractures are a challenge to fix and to get good results. I have seen myself and my colleagues struggling a lot when it comes to fix the intraarticular fractures of lower end of humerus and metaphyseal region. The moment we think of intraarticular fracture; thoughts flows through my mind, (i) Can I fix this fracture rigidly and in anatomic position, (ii) Can I fix it with bicolumnar / bipillar plating, (iii) How good would be my fixation so that I can make elbow mobile as early as possible. This feeling becomes terrifying when it comes to fixation of fractures involving osteoporotic bones, when there is bones loss, when articular cartilage loss is present, and there is a very severe comminution. The patient presenting with bag of bones picture is also terrifying. The thought that run in one's mind is if I would be able to fix these fracture or not, if I would be able to mobilise this patient early so that he/she attains full range of movement. The comminution makes it difficult to open reduce and fix the fracture with simple plating. For the same reason it becomes necessary to convert the distal condylar fragments into one fragment so that the plates or similar kind of hardware can be used with ease.

As that of other surgeons I would be afraid to tackle this type of fracture, as the fixation method available till date like, screw, plates; wires do not hold the bone as rigidly as required. And there are subsequent complications like failure of implants, non-union due to non-rigid fixation. They give either unicortical fixation or fixation that is not so rigid which will make me comfortable to mobilise patient early. This thought process would constantly harass me, when I would take patient of fracture lower end humerus (Intraarticular especially) to operate. But one fine day while operating such case, in the attempt to fix fracture rigidly I tried to fix the fracture of lower end humerus by different method, and this evolved the technique of "TRANSOSSEOUS FIXATION OF FRACTURE BY TENSION BAND TECNIQUE". The moment I was tensioning the stainless steel wire (Tension band wire) from one side, my confidence was growing so much with each turn I was feeling great. At the end of procedure the fixation, stability, rigidity, and bicortical fixation achieved gave me such confidence that, I started to mobilise patient on day 2 of surgery immediately after first wound check (Day 0 - Day of Surgery).

This was the dawn of new technique which I called "TRANSOSSEOUS FIXATION OF FRACTURE BY TENSION BAND TECNIQUE."

With this technique I started fixing fracture of lower end of humerus, fracture involving loss of bones, fractures involving condyle etc. We will discuss all of this in great detail later on. This technique is based on the AO principle of tension band wire where the distraction forces are converted into compressive forces. Here the medial condyle along with the common flexor muscles along with the lateral condyle with common extensor muscles acts as a distracting force.

These forces are converted to compressive forces through a tunnel created transosseously in the lower humeral region. Because the compression achieved with this technique is such immense that early union is expected to happen in the intercondylar region according to the principle of Ilizarov (micromotion at the fracture site causing early union and early mobility).

We propose that this technique could be utilised for the fixation of all fractures which are intraarticular in nature like fracture of upper end of tibia, lower end of femur etc. The immense stability rigidity and early mobility forms the backbone of our technique.

This technique can be utilized instead of interfragmentry fixation of fractures better than using simple screws. The compression achieved by transosseous technique is much superior to interfragmentry fixation.

PRINCIPLES OF TRANSOSSEOUS FIXATION

The transosseous fixation is based on sound principle of physics. It utilises the principle of AO tension band wiring where the distractive forces are converted into compressive forces to achieve union at the fracture sites. Secondly the tensioning of the stainless steel wire done during this procedure which gives adequate compression for the stability and rigidity at the fracture site that allows us early mobility which crates micro-motion at the fracture site leading to early union. The technique proposed by Ilizarov which is worldwide accepted and holds well with our technique also due to early micro-motion at the fracture site. These are the principles on which the transosseous fixation technique is based upon and hold good for the all other metaphyseal intraarticular fractures. A very good bicortical fixation for intraarticular fractures is achieved by this technique.

Added advantage of this technique is that, we can apply the transosseous fixation in more than one plane like in upper end tibia it can be passed in medial to lateral direction and anterior to posterior direction, so we can take care of posterior fragments (posterio medial and posterio lateral) as well.

EPIDEMIOLOGY

Fractures of the elbow constitute about 7% of adult fractures and distal end humerus fractures account for less than half of all elbow fractures [1]. Distal end humerus fractures are relatively uncommon in adults, comprising approximately 2% of all fractures [1] and a third of all humeral fractures [3]. Among patients who sustain a fracture in the distal humerus, there is a bimodal distribution with respect to age and gender, with peaks of incidence in males aged 12 to 19 years and females aged 80 years and over. The vast majority of bicolumnar fractures are displaced [4] and nearly one-fourth are open.

In a ten year prospective study at Edinburgh, United Kingdom (aged 12 years or over), revealed an overall incidence of distal humeral fracture of 5.7 per 100,000 population per year [4]. The respective average ages at fracture for males and females in the Edinburgh series [4] were 36.8 (range 12 to 87 years) and 59.7 years (range 13 to 99 years). The incidence is therefore representative of the pattern of predominantly blunt trauma seen in European populations. The investigators in Finland performed a retrospective review of hospital admission records between 1970 and 1995 and found that the age-adjusted increase in incidence in women older than 60 years had more than doubled [1]

The epidemiology may be different in the United States and in developing countries, due to the greater numbers of severely comminuted open distal humeral fractures produced by blast, gunshot, and industrial injuries in a younger population [5] [6] [7].

There is good evidence that the overall incidence of distal humeral fractures is increasing worldwide [1](8) ,particularly in developed countries. This is mainly due to the rising incidence of osteoporotic fractures from low-energy falls in the elderly. This increase mirrors the changes seen in other regions of the body, most notably in the hip, spine, and distal radius [9]. There is evidence that these fractures are sustained when the arm is axially loaded when the elbow is flexed beyond 90° [10] [11].

ANATOMY OF ELBOW JOINT

In order to understand the transosseous technique; a sound knowledge of lower end humerus anatomy is essential.

Elbow joint is a hinged variety of synovial joint comprised of trochlear process of humerus in articulation with ulnar notch; while capitellum articulates with radial head. It has articular cartilage extending from lower end of humerus covering whole of trochlea, inferior, anteriorly and posteriorly except superiorly where it becomes continuous with metaphysis of humerus. Posteriorly, the cartilage part is well below the olecranon fossa. There is a distinct gap between the articular cartilage and olecranon fossa. The beak of ulna articulates with the olecranon fossa during the complete extension of elbow and sits in it. The cartilage portion of trochlea is below and inferior to the olecranon fossa. Anteriorly and superiorly it is completely covered with cartilage. Superiorly the cartilage part where it mingles with the bony part of humerus there is a small depression where coronoid process of ulna comes and rests in full flexion. The medial epicondyle is attached with medial the condyle of humerus. Between the medial epicondyle and articular cartilage of trochlear process is a place where there is no cartilage. This landmark is very important in our technique of transosseous fixation because while placing the tunnel we place our tunnel very low in this area so that it is just above the cartilaginous process and we don't involve the articular cartilage. Medially just below the epicondyle and above articular cartilage we place our initial stainless steel guide wire or a K wire along with washer. There is good amount of space which is extraarticular between medial epicondyle and common flexor origin where we can safely place our implant.

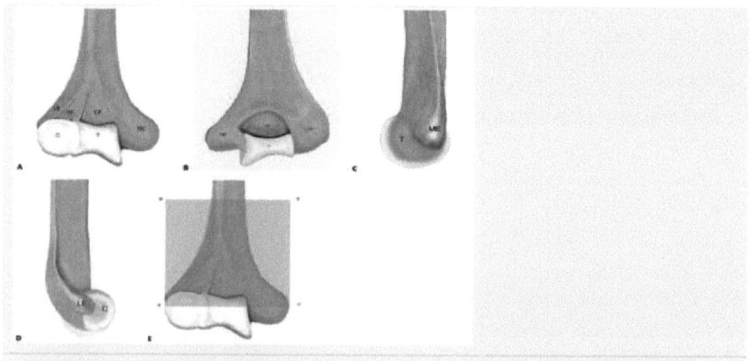

FIGURE 29-4 The bony landmarks of the distal humerus. A. Anterior view. B. Posterior view. C. Medial view. D. Lateral view. E. The hypothetical boundaries of the distal humeral metaphysis (A,B,C,D). T, trochlea; C, capitellum; ME, medial epicondyle; LE, lateral epicondyle; CF, coronoid fossa; RF, radial fossa; OF, olecranon fossa.

COURTESY ROCKWOOD AND GREEN 7TH EDITION

Lateral part of trochlea blends with the capitellum on the lateral aspect. Capitellum is also covered anteriorly, superiorly and inferiorly with articular cartilage. It has a grove on the anterior superior surface where the cartilage ends and metaphyseal bone starts. This fossa is called as a radial fossa where radial head comes and sits in the full flexion. Lateral most part of a capitellum is lateral condyle of the humerus which is again free from cartilage. This is also a place where we place our implants in transosseous fixation. Also in this part common extensor group of muscles takes its origin while the lateral part bends with the lateral column of the humerus. At distal end of humerus medial and lateral collateral ligaments attaches on medial and lateral aspect just below where column or supracondylar ridges end.

Inferior part of the joint is formed by the ulna and radius medially and laterally respectively. Ulna which is beak shaped and which has articular surface which articulate with the trochlea of humerus and has an olecranon process and coronoid process. Olecranon process sits in the olecranon fossa posteriorly on extension and coronoid process sits in coronoid fossa anteriorly on full flexion. Laterally the radial head is fully covered with cartilage and articulates with the capitellum of humerus. The medial part of the radial head articulates with proximal end of ulna in radial notch. Whole of this joint along with the cartilage margin is covered with capsule of the elbow joint. The details and thorough knowledge of the joint anatomy is essential to place the transosseous tunnels very near to the articulating surface of the joint. The medial part of trochlear surface is inferiorly placed as compared to lateral side so while placing the tunnel from medial side wire has to be directed superiorly and laterally so that it doesn't enter the joint.

The distal humerus consists of the expanded portion of the metaphysis, including the joint surfaces for articulation with the corresponding surfaces of the proximal ulna and radial head. They are usually considered to be metaphyseal if the major fragments are located within a hypothetical square, with sides equal the widest portion of the distal metaphysis.

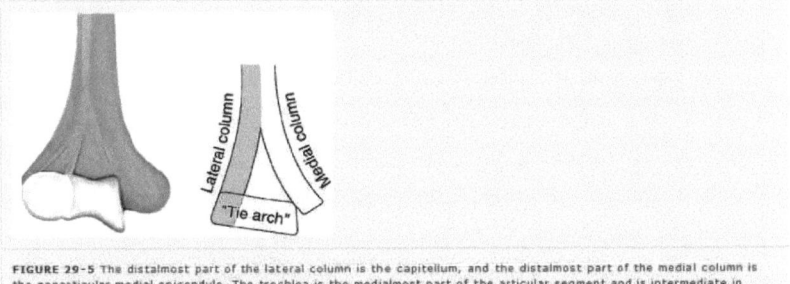

FIGURE 29-5 The distalmost part of the lateral column is the capitellum, and the distalmost part of the medial column is the nonarticular medial epicondyle. The trochlea is the medialmost part of the articular segment and is intermediate in position between the medial epicondyle and capitellum. The articular segment functions architecturally as a âCœtie arch.â€

COURTESY ROCKWOOD AND GREEN 7TH EDITION

The ulnotrochlear and radiocapitellar joints are functionally independent joints. The flexion and extension of the elbow occurs at a uniaxial ulnotrochlear joint. The trochlea forms a pulley and has an articular arc of 270° with medial and lateral eminences, with an intervening sulcus, which articulates with the semilunar notch of the proximal ulna. The eminences of the pulley provide medial and lateral stability to the simple hinge joint but there could be up to 5° of varus or valgus laxity in response to applied force during movement of elbow joint. In contrast, the radiocapitellar joint is mechanically linked to the distal radioulnar joint, and both subserve forearm rotational movements, independent of the position of the ulnotrochlear joint. The pulley-like trochlea forms the central articulating axis of the ulnotrochlear joint and acts as "tie-arch" between the two thickened condensations of bone along the medial and lateral epicondylar ridges of the distal humeral metaphysis, which constitute the two columns of the elbow.

The crux of treatment of distal end humerus fracture is mechanical stability by re-creating this triangle of stability. The columns and the trochlea are the strongest part which is the place where internal fixation plate or screws can be applied.

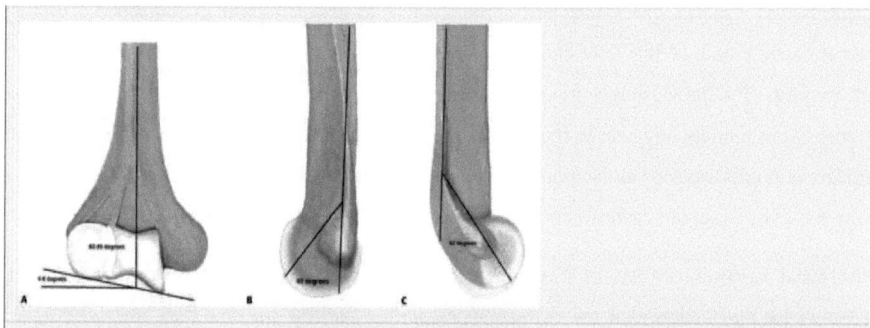

FIGURE 29-6 The joint surface to shaft axis is 4Å° to 8Å° of valgusâ€"the A-carrying angle (A). The articular segment juts forward from the line of the shaft at 40Å° and functions architecturally as the tie arch at the point of maximum column divergence distally. It is important to note that the medial epicondyle is on the projected axis of the shaft, whereas the lateral epicondyle is projected slightly forward from the axis (B,C).

COURTESY ROCKWOOD AND GREEN 7TH EDITION

The normal carrying angle of the elbow is produced by the valgus offset of the longitudinal axis of the trochlea, with respect to the longitudinal axis of the humerus. The trochlear axis is also externally rotated between 3 and 8 degrees with respect to a line connecting the medial and the lateral epicondyles, and both the trochlea and capitellum project forward at an angle of approximately 40 degrees from the long axis of the humerus.

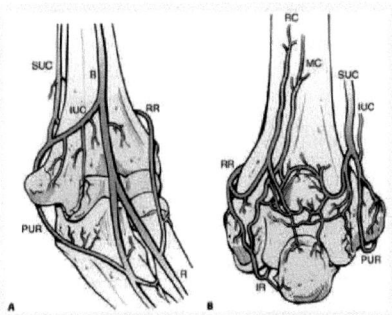

FIGURE 29-12 The blood supply of the distal humerus. **A.** Anterior view. **B.** Posterior view. *SUC*, superior ulnar collateral artery; *B*, brachial artery; *IUC*, inferior ulnar collateral artery; *RR*, radial recurrent artery; *PUR*, posterior ulnar recurrent artery; *R*, radial artery; *RC*, radial collateral artery; *MC*, middle collateral artery; *IR*, interosseous recurrent artery. (Redrawn after Yamaguchi K, Sweet FA, Bindra R, et al. The extraosseous and intraosseous arterial anatomy of the adult elbow. *J Bone Joint Surg Am* 1997;79:1653â€"1662, with permission.)

COURTESY ROCKWOOD AND GREEN 7TH EDITION

The blood supply to the distal end of humerus has derived from the brachial artery with its branches along with the recurrent branches from radial and ulnar artery, laterally and medially respectively.

MECHANISM OF INJURY

Most low-energy distal humeral fractures are produced from simple domestic falls in middle-aged and elderly females in which the elbow is either struck directly or axially loaded in a fall onto the outstretched hand [4]. Road-traffic accidents and sport are a more common cause of injury in younger males. A higher proportion of these injuries are open fractures and these patients often have other injuries. In the Edinburgh series, 17% of patients had other orthopaedic injuries and 5% sustained multisystem injuries [4]. There is evidence that these fractures are sustained when the arm is axially loaded when the elbow is flexed beyond 90° [12].

Most of the patients with intraarticular injuries were patients of a road traffic accident who sustained injuries due to direct fall on their elbow, while the older patients with osteoporotic bones sustained intraarticular fractures due to fall on outstretched hand and axial loading.

Most of the fractures were of comminuted types were found in older age group patients than younger ones. The patients with bone loss were found in the older age group patients. Some of the young patients who suffered intraarticular fractures were working at the construction site and their injuries were due to fall from height on an outstretched hand. Open fractures were found in younger age group patients than in older age group patients.

Cases of direct trauma to the elbow due to blow from a stick were also found. These injuries usually comprised of closed and comminuted fractures. Fall from trees or height on an outstretched hand were also the cause for some of the fractures. Knowing the mechanism or the injury is very important in dealing with these fractures as usually the fractures due to trivial trauma are difficult to treat due to poor quality of the bone, while injuries due to direct trauma are open and difficult to deal again.

CLINICAL EVALUATION

- Patients with this type of fractures usually presents with degree of swelling and displacement, rendering landmarks difficult to palpate. However, an equilateral triangle maintains the normal relationship of the olecranon, medial, and lateral condyles.

- Swelling, ecchymosis, crepitus with difficulty in range of motion and gross instability may be present, although this is highly suggestive of fracture, no attempt should be made to elicit it because neurovascular compromise may result.

- Patients with open fractures will present with wound which could be classified on the basis of Gustilo Anderson open injury grading and can be further treated accordingly

- It's very essential for clinical and medico legal aspect to check the neurovascular status of upper extremity as the sharp, fractured end of the proximal fragment may impinge or contuse the brachial artery, median nerve, or radial nerve.

- Serial neurovascular examinations with compartment pressure monitoring may be necessary with massive swelling, cubital fossa swelling may result in vascular impairment or the development of a volar compartment syndrome resulting in Volkmann ischemia.

- The patients with this injuries presents with severe deformity and usually with varus angulation of upper extremity.

- The local examination would reveal a bluish discoloration of the elbow, swelling of the elbow and in open fractures contamination and bleeding of the joint with or without bone loss.

- There would be immense tenderness, local rise of temperature, crepitus, and deformity of the upper extremity.

- Sometimes there would be blister formations, posteriorly and anteriorly on the elbow joint.

- In open fractures comminuted bone fragments, loose bone pieces, foreign bodies, blood vessels, torn muscles, disrupted and rough skin edges would be found at the injury site.

- In young patients and those with the road traffic accidents, it is mandatory to first clinically examine the patient for the vital systems like the cardiovascular, brain, respiratory, urinary and to rule out life threatening abdominal injuries.

- In road traffic accidents, the vital organ examination and resuscitation of the patient takes priority in treatment over the elbow fractures

- The neurovascular examination and the examination of the rest of the joint of extremity are of immense importance.

RADIOLOGICAL EVALUATION

- Standard anteroposterior (AP), lateral and oblique views of the elbow should be obtained. Traction radiographs are better for preoperative planning as they delineate the fracture pattern very well.

- In non-displaced fractures, an anterior or posterior "fat pad sign" may be present on the lateral radiograph, representing displacement of the adipose layer overlying the joint capsule in the presence of effusion or heamarthrosis.

- The normal condylar shaft angle on lateral radiographs will be decreased in the minimally displaced fractures. (Normal condylar shaft angle of 40 degrees).

- Because intercondylar fractures are much more common than supracondylar fractures in adults, the AP (or oblique) radiograph should be scrutinized for evidence of a vertical split in the intercondylar region of the distal humerus.

- The standard AP and lateral X-ray of the patient should be thoroughly evaluated. In AP X-ray, one should look for the intraarticular extension of the fracture, the amount of comminution, the amount of bone loss, the fracture pattern, the geometry of the fracture can be evaluated very well, while in the lateral X-ray, again the amount of displacement, the amount of comminution, the extension of the fracture fragment, the pieces of the fractured bone and to some extent the rotation of the fracture fragment can be evaluated very well. Once this is evaluated in a proper way once can think of evaluation of both the lateral and medial pillars and evaluation of the olecranon fossa. One can also evaluate to certain extent the hardware to be used to fix these fractures

- The thorough evaluation of low intraarticular fractures is essential in placing the transosseous tunnels in the lower segment very close to the joint. The comminution if any in the condylar region should be evaluated seriously in the AP and the lateral view X-Ray as we are going to place all hardware there.

- The bag of bone picture seen in the X-ray of the elbow of elderly patients with osteoporosis should be seen very seriously as there is lot of bone loss and lot of cartilage loss in these patients, also the simple looking X-ray, has lot of bone pieces and it is a challenge to fix.

- A better view of the fracture fragments, cartilage, joint surface and bone loss can be evaluated by modern days CT scan of the elbow with 2D and 3D reconstruction. If facilities available the re-construction of the fractured part and stabilization and fixation of the fragments can be done in the radiological room. The step could be recorded, the fragments could be labelled and the implant fixed in anatomical position could be done by navigation along with CT.

- It is a dictum nowadays to do CT elbow along with the X-rays for all patients with intraarticular fractures.

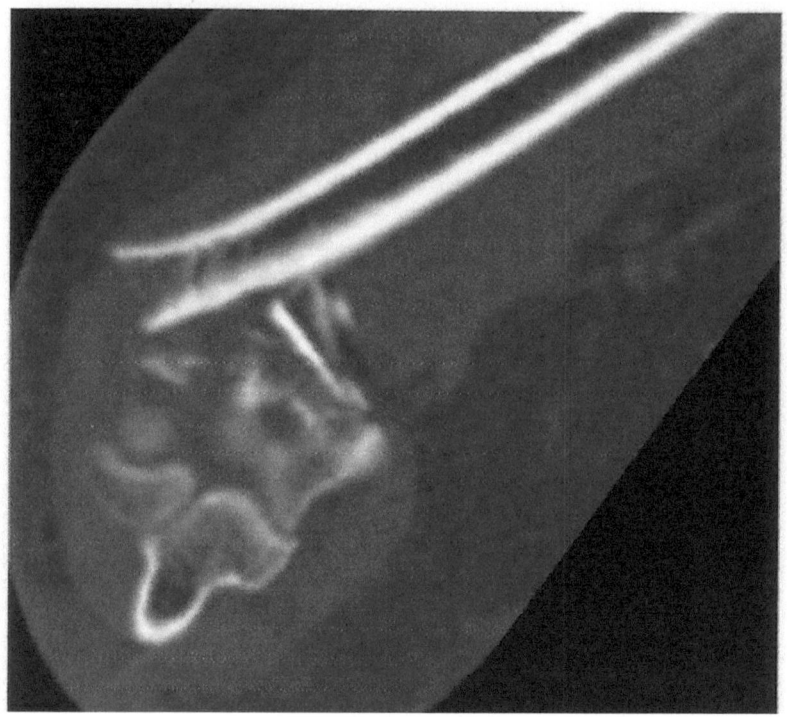

CT scan elbow

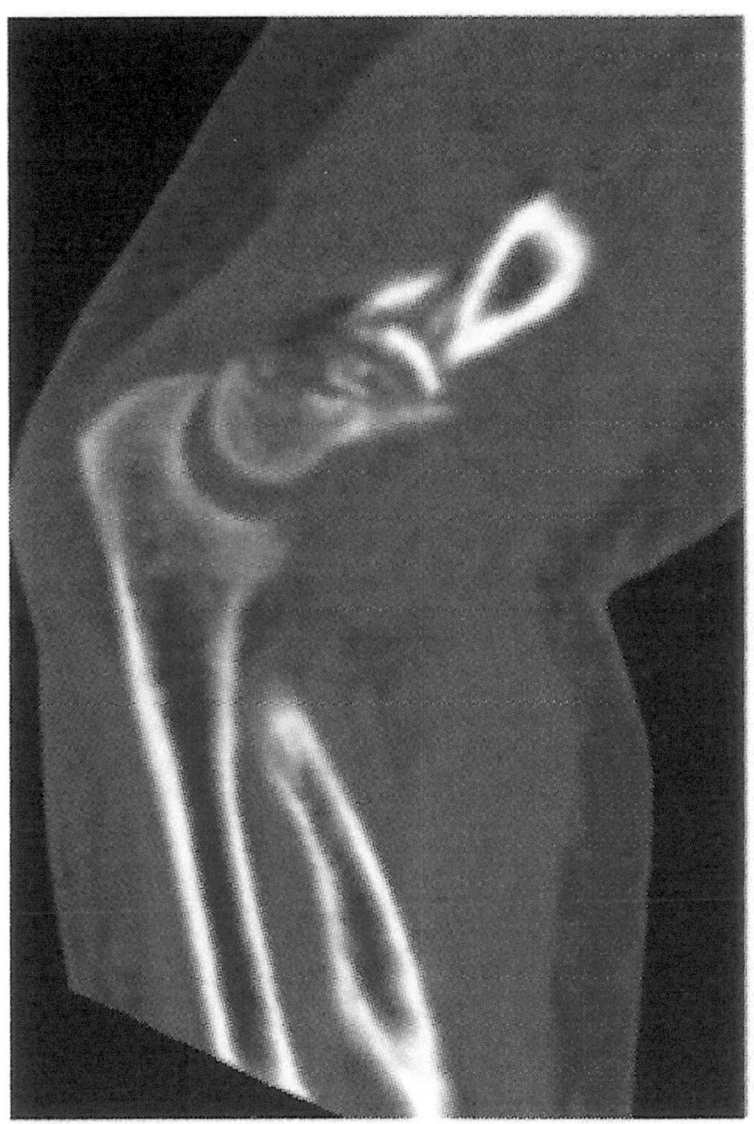

CT Scan Elbow

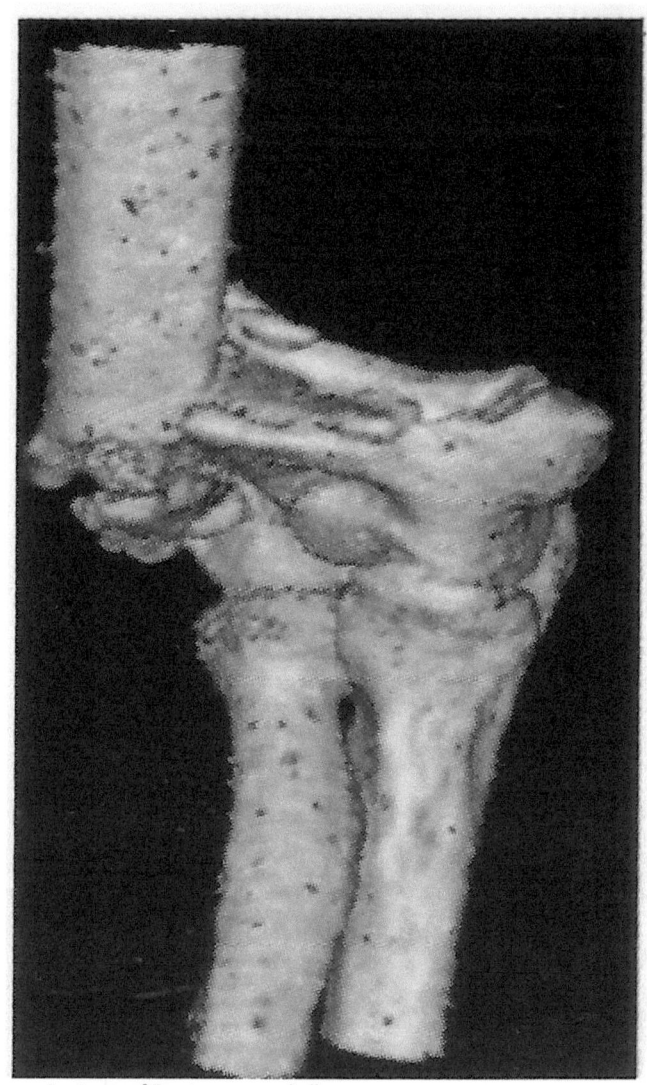

Anatomy of Fracture around elbow

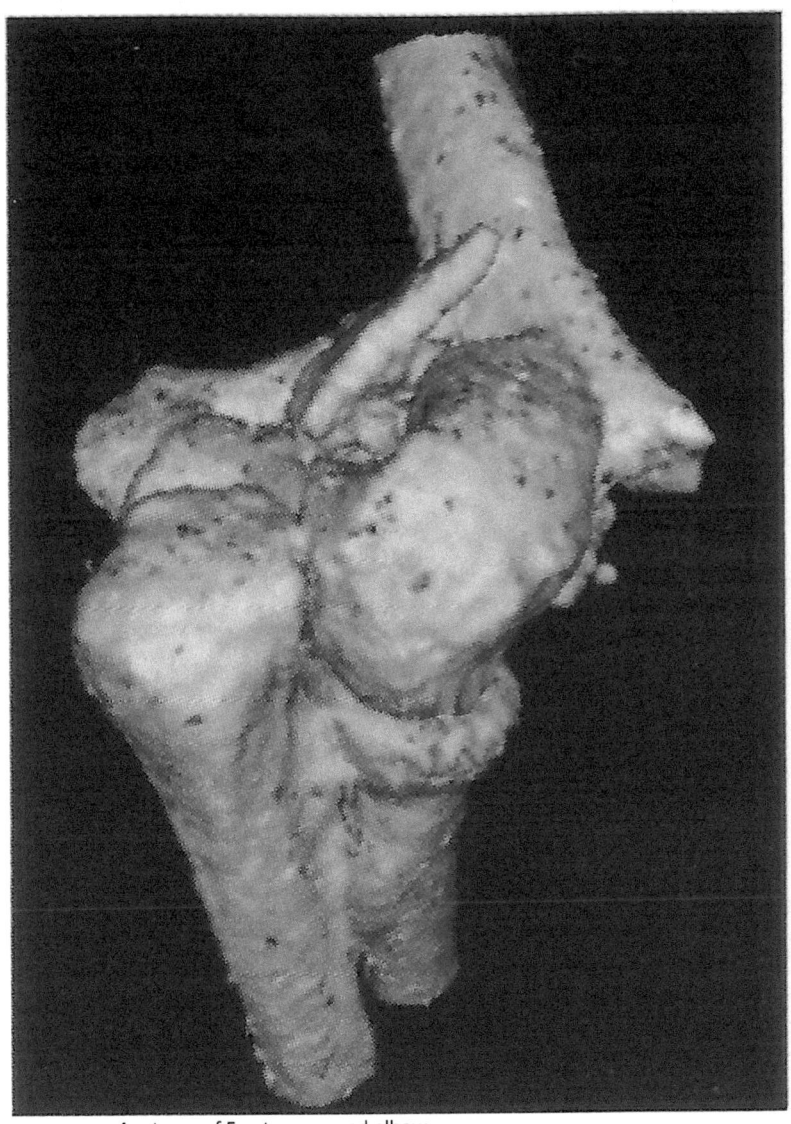

Anatomy of Fracture around elbow

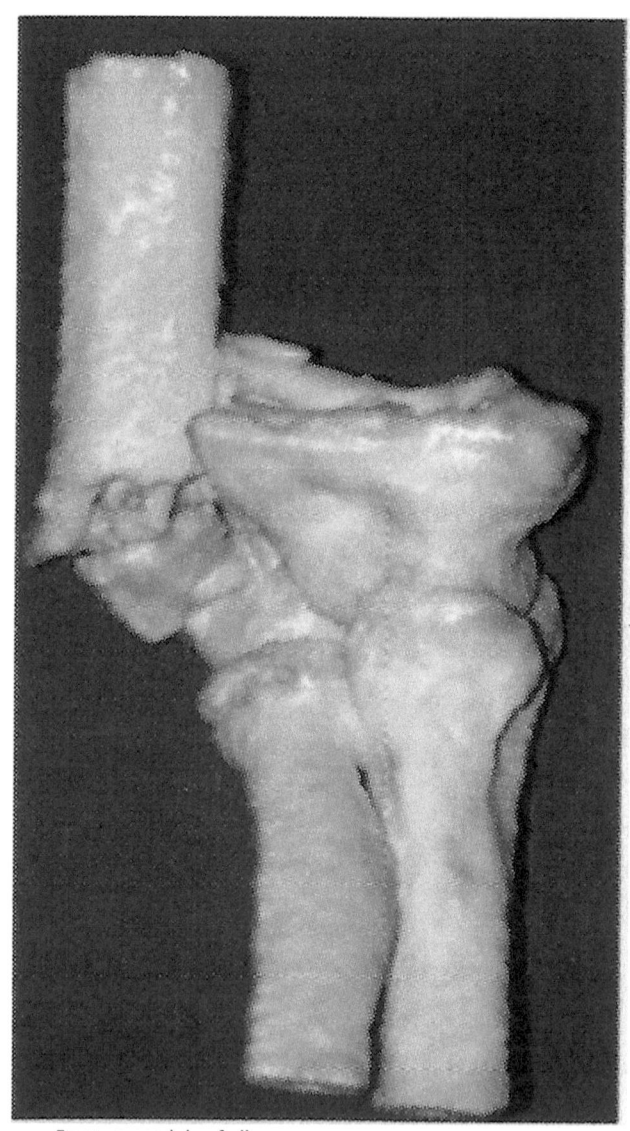

Fracture module of elbow

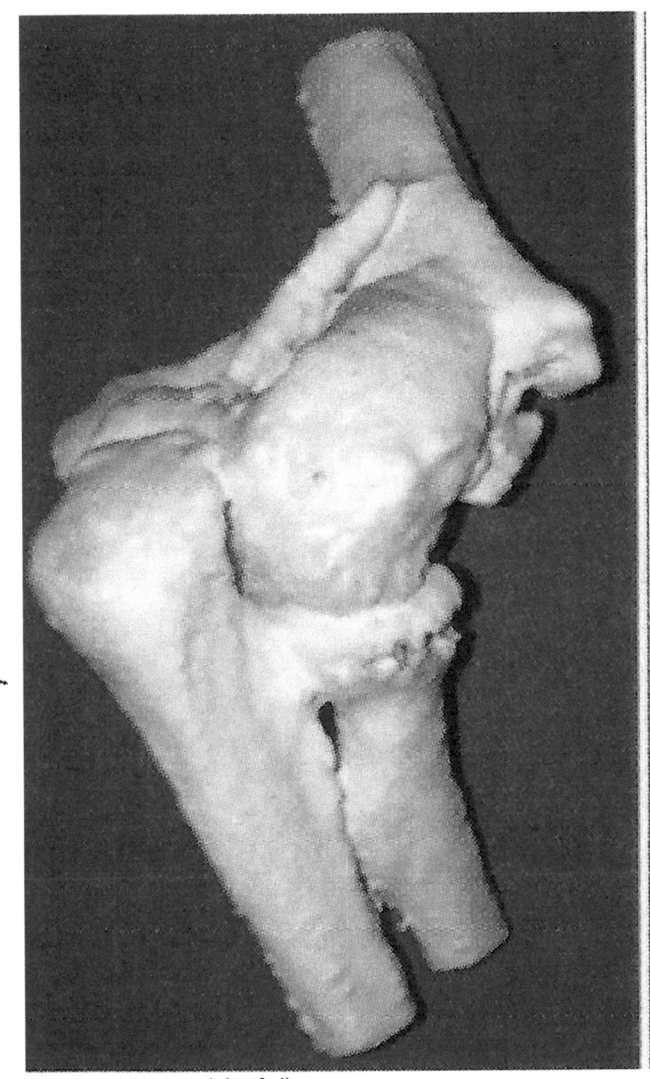

Fracture module of elbow

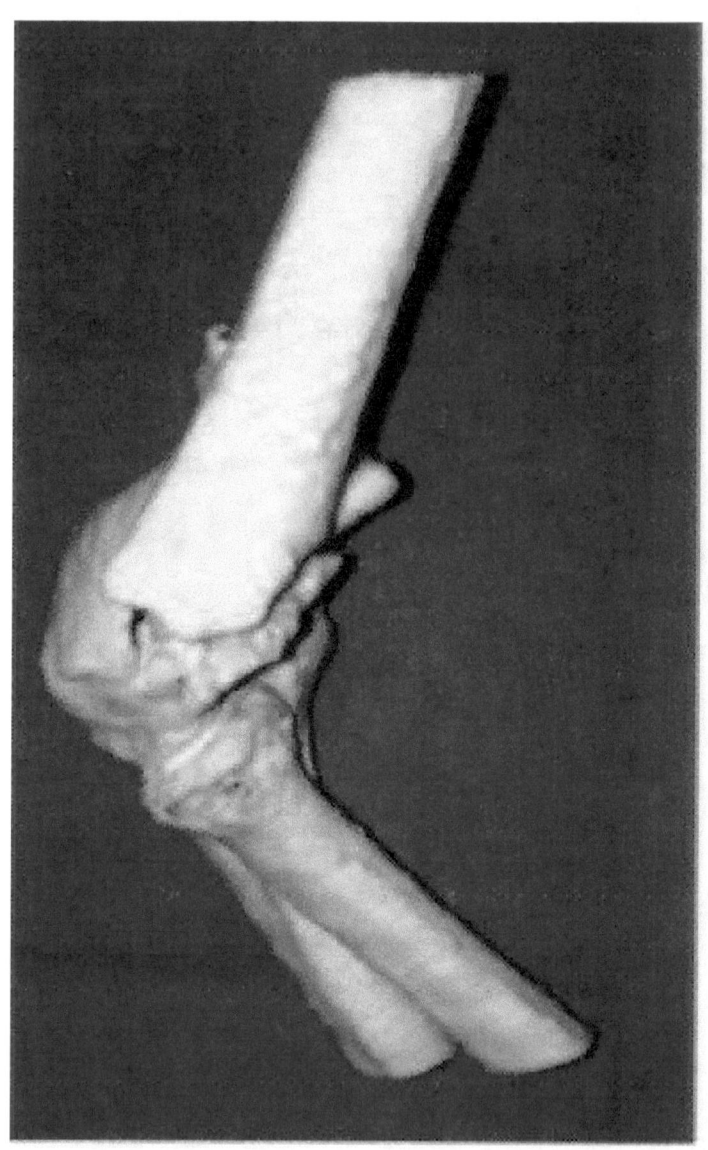

Fracture module of elbow

CLASSIFICATIONS

Descriptive:

- Supracondylar fractures

    o Extension-type
    o Flexion-type
- Transcondylar fractures
- Intercondylar fractures
- Condylar fractures
- Capitellum fractures
- Trochlea fractures
- Lateral epicondylar fractures
- Medial epicondylar fractures
- Fractures of the supracondylar process

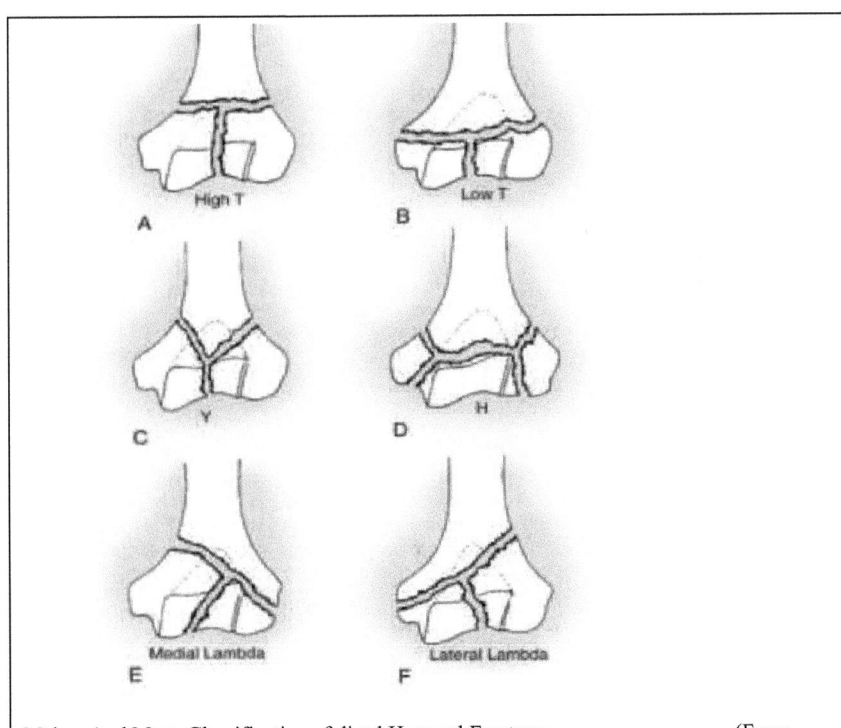

Mehne And Matta Classification of distal Humeral Fractures   (From
Jupiter JB: Internal fixation for fracture about the elbow, Op Tech Orthop4:34, 1994)

Riseborough and Radin Classification

Type I: Non-displaced

Type II: Slight displacement with no rotation between the condylar fragments

Type III: Displacement with rotation

Type IV: Severe comminution of the articular surface

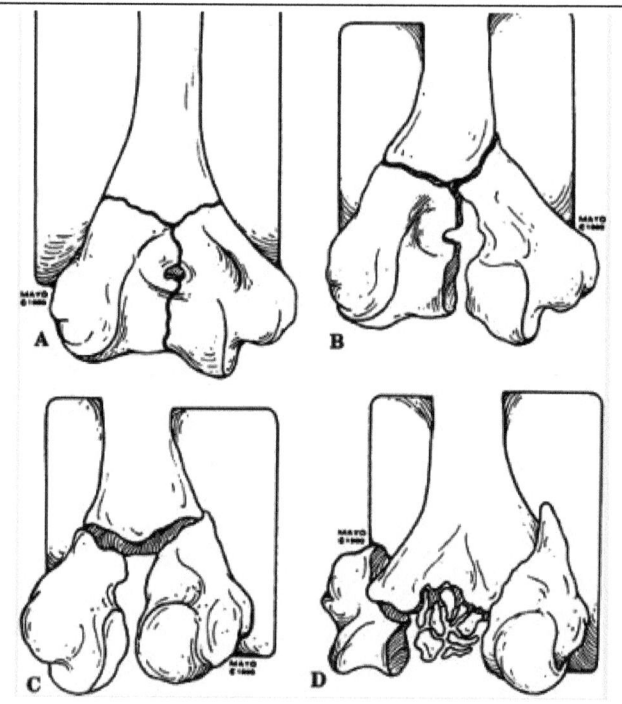

Riseborough and Radin Classification
(A) Type I Undisplaced Condylar # of the elbow (B) type II Displaced but not rotated condylar fracture (C) Type III Displaced and rotated condylar Fracture (D) Type IV Displaced, Rotated and comminuted condylar fracture. (From Bryan R S, Fractures about the Elbow in adults, AAOS Instr Course Lect 1981; 30:200-223)

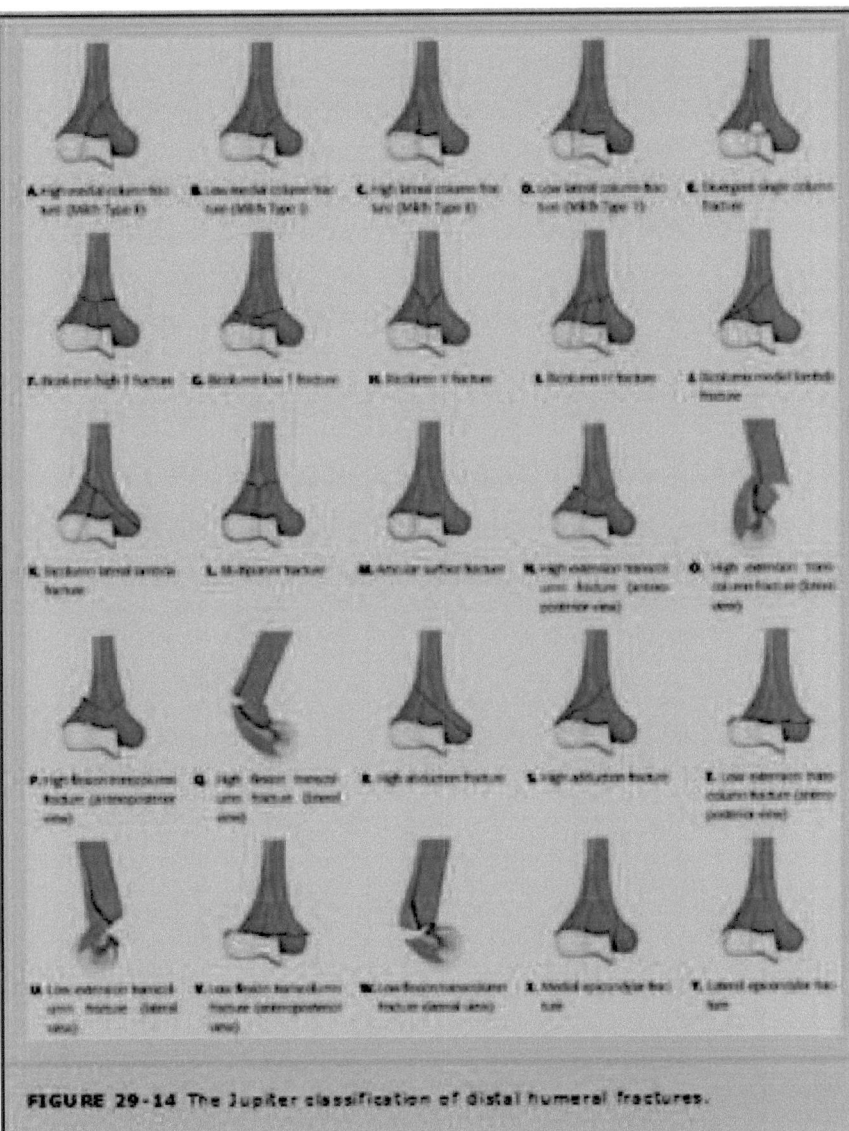

FIGURE 29-14 The Jupiter classification of distal humeral fractures.

SURGICAL APPROACHES FOR FIXATION

The Fixation of intraarticular fractures of lower end of humerus is done by posterior approach, using osteotomy or non-osteotomy method. Let us discuss first with osteotomy approach.

Posterior approach with olecranon osteotomy:

Fixation for fractures of lower end of humerus; intraarticular can be visualised very well by this approach with osteotomy. Osteotomy can be of two types; intraarticular type and extraarticular type. Both of these can be chevron type or direct in variety. By this approach the total view of articular surface of lower end of humerus can be done along with visualisation of posterior part, inferior part and anterior part of articular surface. Medial condyle lateral condyle, olecranon fossa and both pillars of distal end of humerus can be visualised directly without the help of image intensifier. It becomes very easy to place tunnels through the bone without the help of image intensifier. Secondly the placement of plates along the columns can be done easily by this approach. Screws and implants can be placed and can be checked whether the both cortices involved or not by this approach.

Procedure:

Patient put in lateral position with tourniquet in place. A support frame applied for the elbow holding on the respective side. Incision over the posterior aspect of elbow extending 5 to 7 cm above and below olecranon process tip. It is deepened inside after subcutaneous dissection and the triceps is well visualised and separated posterior and the ulna nerve is identified and isolated, retracted medially by looping it in an infant feeding tube. Then osteotomy site is marked (intra or extraarticular) on the bone, two third of osteotomy done with the help of saw and remaining one third with the help of sharp osteotome. Damage to the articular surface is prevented by keeping a haemostat in the joint and then osteotomy is completed. Once the osteotomy is complete the triceps along with bone fragment lifted up and incision is taken along the two pillars and the total triceps is elevated from the posterior aspect with the help of periosteum. Some of the periosteum along the medial and lateral pillars has to be dealt with electrocautery so that we can place plate and screws along the medial and lateral pillar without difficulty. For the ant visualisation of articular cartilage the elbow is flexed beyond 90 degree and this gives clear visualisation of all surfaces and pillars of the distal humerus. This completes the posterior approach with osteotomy.

Schematic Diagram of right olecranon osteotomy

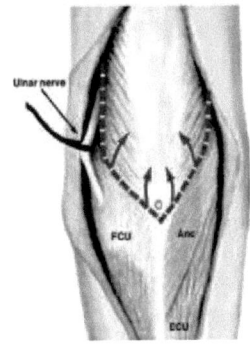

Preparation of site

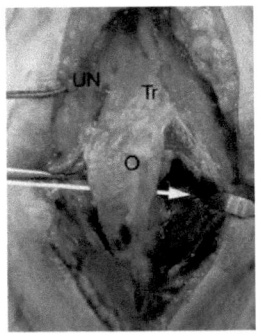

Performing the chevron osteotomy

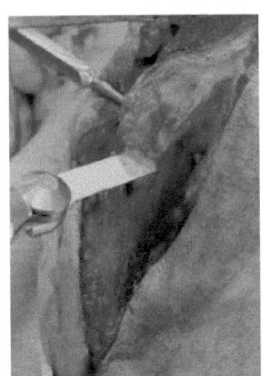

Completion of osteotomy with osteotome

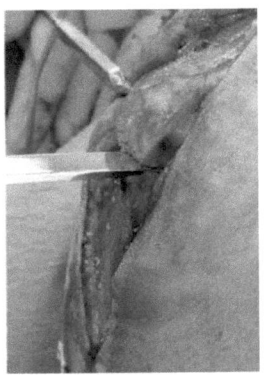

Retraction of olecranon with towel forcep

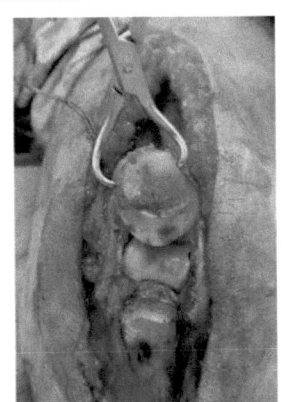

Final Fixation with TBW

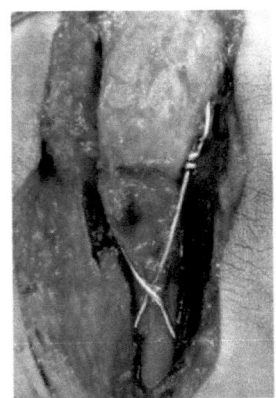

Drawback of this approach

1. A new fracture is created and to fix this an extra implant required to fix this so lot of hardware seen in elbow region
2. Complications of this hardware
3. Complication of the new fracture like non-union, malunion can happen

Non osteotomy approach:

Extensile elbow approach in which there are three varieties like triceps splitting, triceps reflecting and triceps detaching approach (By Brian Morrey). Authors preferred approach is extensile triceps reflecting among nonosteotomy approaches. Incision over the posterior aspect of elbow 5 cm above and below olecranon process tip. It is deepened inside after subcutaneous dissection and the triceps is well visualised and separated posteriorly and the ulnar nerve is identified and isolated and retracted medially by looping it in an infant feeding tube.

With 11 number blade sharp dissection done over proximal ulna from medial to the lateral side so that the periosteum along with the insertion of the triceps is carried out in one unit fully and lifted completely from medial to the lateral aspect. As we go on lifting it laterally the entire proximal portion of the ulna along with olecranon process becomes totally bare. The periosteum reflection is continued below and muscle along with the periosteum is reflected from the bone inferiorly around 5 to 7 cm such that it reflected completely as a single unit. In this way a continuous tissue layer is created along the tissues which are inferiorly attached on the ulna along with triceps tendon. Laterally this incision is completed by dissecting tricep anconeus flap. By this approach a complete exposure of the both columns along with both condyles and articular surfaces is achieved.

The anterior portion of the articular surface can be visualized by hyper flexing the elbow beyond 90°. While closure the tricep tendon has to be drilled and fixed over the olecranon process, by non-absorbable sutures.

Schematic Presentation of triceps reflecting

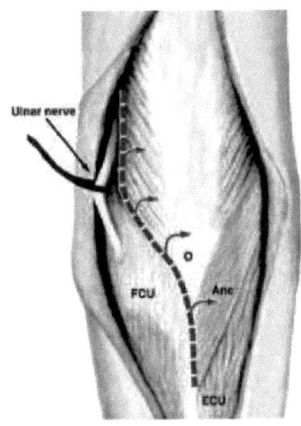 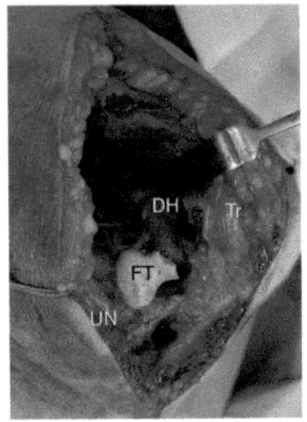

FIGURE 29-10 The triceps-reflecting (Morrey) approach. **A.** Schematic diagram of the approach in a right elbow with the patient in a lateral decubitus position (*FCU*, flexor carpi ulnaris; *ECU*, extensor carpi ulnaris; *Anc*, anconeus). **B.** Intraoperative view of the approach (*Tr*, triceps; *FT*, fractured trochlea; *UN*, ulnar nerve; *DH*, distal humerus).

Advantages of this approach:

No new fracture created

No issues of non-union or malunion as no osteotomy done here

Faster recovery

Drawbacks:

Triceps tendon ruptures intra-operatively and postoperatively

Myositis ossificans

Extensive nature of the exposure

Lateral column visualisation slightly difficult

Good surgical skills required for this approach

Other approaches

Triceps-Splitting

The triceps-splitting approach fashioning is a direct midline posterior split in the triceps developed in an attempt to overcome the morbidity associated with the use of olecranon osteotomy [13] [14] [15] [16] [17]. A thin wafer of bone may be detached from the olecranon at the level of the triceps insertion and reflect the triceps insertion off the olecranon and proximal ulna medially and laterally [16].

The access to the joint surfaces anteriorly can be improved by flexing the elbow and grasping and posteriorly retracting the olecranon with reduction. Some authors have reported a better functional outcome with this approach as it does not appear to be detrimental to elbow function [18] and reduces the risk of later hardware complications, encountered with the use of an olecranon osteotomy [18] [19], others have reported the converse [20]. Another major advantage of this approach is that it allows greater intraoperative flexibility, because either internal fixation or total elbow arthroplasty (TER) can be performed. The major drawback of the triceps-splitting approach is the theoretical risk of postoperative detachment of the tendon from the proximal ulna, though this has not been reported to date. Care must be taken not to split muscle more proximally as it could damage radial nerve [19].

Triceps-Reflecting

This approach was developed for insertion of a TER, without the requirement to fully detach the triceps insertion, in patients with degenerative joint disease [21] [22]. It can also be used to treat a distal humerus fracture because the distal portions of both columns and the articular surfaces are excised, creating a sloppy working space, in which the components of the elbow replacement can be inserted. This approach gives limited exposure to the lateral column so less often used for the open reduction and internal fixation of distal end humerus fractures. The whole of the triceps is reflected as a continuous cuff of tissue, from medial to lateral. The medial aspect of the triceps is sharply reflected off the proximal ulna at its insertion, taking care to only continue dissection until adequate exposure of the joint has been obtained. As with the triceps-splitting approach, careful repair of the triceps tendon through drill holes is required to reduce the risk of postoperative tendon pull-off.

Variations of this approach:

- As originally described there is a risk of ulnar nerve palsy from retraction during surgery [21]. To protect against this the triceps may be split so that 75% of the muscle lies laterally and 25% medially [23]. The triceps is then reflected laterally as for the standard technique. The ulnar nerve and its blood supply are protected from traction injury by the medial triceps during surgery.
- A wafer of bone carrying the triceps insertion may be detached, to facilitate later closure. The triceps is then reflected laterally as a "tricipito-anconeus flap" to provide exposure of the lateral column [24].
- The paratricipital approach, originally described by Alonso-Llames [25] has been adapted for use in transcolumnar and simple bicolumnar fractures [26]. Through a single posterior incision, exposure of the medial and lateral columns is made by separate medial and lateral paratricipital incisions, with minimal retraction of the triceps.
- The triceps may be reflected from lateral to medial (extended Kocher approach). This approach has seldom been used for fractures of the distal humerus.
- Morrey has further modified his original approach for non-union surgery, where the distal humeral articular surface is to be excised to insert a hinged TER [27]. If the patient has undergone previous surgery, detachment of the triceps insertion from the ulna may be inadvisable, in view of the greater risk of subsequent triceps pull-off. The triceps is therefore not reflected off the ulna and more limited lateral reflection of the triceps, sufficient only to allow excision of the distal humerus, is performed. The residual distal humerus can be delivered into the wound either medial or lateral to the triceps insertion, to allow insertion of the humeral component. The proximal ulna can be exposed by rotating it externally or internally to facilitate insertion of the ulnar component.

Triceps-Detaching Approaches

The triceps-reflecting anconeus pedicle approach (TRAP approach) raises the triceps and anconeus as a continuous flap, through a single posterior incision using separate lateral Kocher and medial approaches [28]. The entire triceps and anconeus are then detached and retracted proximally. A very meticulous repair at the end of surgery is required at the end of the procedure. The excellent exposure of the whole of the distal humerus provided by this approach, which allows either elbow fixation or replacement techniques to be performed easily. The major disadvantage of this procedure is that the triceps is completely detached from the ulna, and is therefore at risk of later detachment or weakness.

Medial Approach

Medial approaches are used when limited access is required to treat single medial column, medial epicondylar, or trochlear fractures. Complex trochlear or capitellar-trochlear fractures can be treated with combined medial and lateral approaches through separate skin incisions. However, this is to be discouraged, as later reconstructive surgery is made more difficult.

The entire medial column of the distal humerus can be accessed through a medial approach. This diverges from the humeral shaft at a 40 degrees angle. The medial epicondyle provides the origin for the flexor muscles of the forearm, and for the anterior and posterior bundles of the medial collateral ligament (MCL). This approach gives limited access to the trochlea and coronoid fossa which lies anterosuperior to it. Alternatively, an osteotomy of the medial epicondyle, with reflection of the common flexor origin, may provide enhanced access to the trochlea.

Lateral Approach

High transcolumnar, simple lateral column, and capitellar fractures can be treated by proximal extension of the Kocher approach [29]. It may be used to gain access to the lateral column of the distal humerus. A posterolateral skin incision, raising a lateral skin flap is preferable to a direct lateral approach, if there is concern that the approach may not give enough access. With the use of this posterior skin incision, extension into either a posterior approach or a separate medial approach can be easily undertaken. Proximally, the triceps is peeled off the lateral intermuscular septum, carefully identifying and preserving the posterior antebrachial cutaneous and radial nerves. Lifting up the triceps from the lateral intermuscular septum allows direct access to the posterolateral surface of the lateral column along with direct visualization of brachioradialis and extensor carpi radialis longus muscles origin on lateral supracondylar ridge. These can be detached from the lateral epicondyle to provide exposure of the lateral aspect of the elbow joint. Exposure of the posterior aspect of the posterior column can also be gained to internally fix capitellar fractures. The lateral epicondyle may be osteotomized or fractured as a result of injury, providing an improved portal of access to the lateral side of the joint for reconstruction[31]. The lateral epicondyle is smaller than its medial counterpart and serves as origin for the lateral collateral ligament, which blends with the common extensor origin and the annular ligament. The anterior fibres of the lateral collateral ligament insert on the supinator crest of the proximal ulna. The common extensor muscle mass takes its origin from the lateral epicondyle, posterior to the radial part of the lateral collateral ligament. The lateral column diverges from the humeral shaft at the same level as the medial column. The proximal part of this column is hard and predominantly cortical bone, whereas the distal half of the lateral column is largely cancellous. The capitellum consists of a 180 degrees hemisphere of cartilage, which faces directly anteriorly. Its rotational centre is displaced between 1 and 2 cm anterior to the axis of the humeral shaft axis, to align it with the trochlea, and allow the radius and ulna to flex and extend coaxially.

Anterior Approach

Anterior approaches are infrequently used in adult distal humeral fracture treatment (32,33). This approach could be used for vascular access if there is a significant injury to the brachial artery at the level of the fracture. The intervening flexor muscles and neurovascular structures, which are at risk of injury and poor access to the medial and lateral columns is the reason why this approach is not used for reconstruction purpose. The two corresponding anterior recesses are the coronoid and radial fossae, which accommodate the coronoid process and radial head during elbow flexion. The fossae are separated by a longitudinal ridge of bone that continues distally as the lateral eminence of the trochlea.

OPERATIVE TECHNIQUES

Patient is given lateral position after appropriate anaesthesia. Tourniquet is applied high in the arm. In lateral position a well-padded support is kept such that the forearm hangs beyond the lateral support so that it can be easily manipulated. A preoperative antibiotic of choice is transfused before the start of surgery, patient is painted and draped after scrubbing as per the standard protocol. If required the graft area is also painted and draped (Iliac crest). A posterior approach with an osteotomy planned. 10 cm long incision well beyond elbow joint over the ulna is taken. Layer by layer dissection is done. Ulnar nerve is identified and medially dissected and taken well beyond medial epicondyle. While doing ulnar nerve dissection take care that some soft tissue remains attached and nerve is not completely stripped of the soft tissue. Don't make the nerve nude. According to personal choice one might use rubber catheter to retract the nerve medially. But I personally don't use rubber catheter as I believe excessive traction with rubber catheter even leads to neuropraxia kind of injuries to the nerve. I personally avoid traction injuries by dissecting the nerve proximally more and nerve stays in position beyond medial epicondyle without any strain or stretch.

Once the nerve is out of picture attention is focussed in doing an ulnar osteotomy. A chevron osteotomy performed as planned after marking osteotomy site on ulna with the help of electrocautery. Once the osteotomy is started two third of bone is cut by saw and remaining cuts made with sharp osteotome. In order to prevent damage to the articular cartilage a haemostat kept in the elbow joint from medial to lateral side. While doing osteotomy osteotome hits on the haemostat and articular cartilage injury is prevented. Once the osteotomy is completed the bone along with the triceps attached with it is pulled upwards and sharp dissection done along medal side over supracondylar region. Muscles attached to the posterior aspect are elevated with the periosteum elevator from medial to lateral side. The lateral supracondylar ridge along with lateral condyle the soft tissues are sharply cut and elevated proximally. The muscles also attached on the posterior aspect are lifted upwards. After the completion of this process, the piece of olecranon bone with attached muscles is lifted upwards and this gives a complete visualisation of articular surfaces of elbow joint, the medial and lateral condyle, the medial and lateral columns and olecranon fossa and posterior surface of the humerus. The visualisation of anterior articular surface of the lower end of humerus is possible when flexion more than 90 degree is done at the elbow joint. At this stage a thorough wash is given so that all the fractures are better seen. Thorough wash also cleans up the clots on the fracture surface and better visualisation of fracture anatomy is possible. Now the geometry of the fracture is studied and all fragments at the fracture site thoroughly identified. Loose pieces of the bone and cartilage are identified and kept safely on the table. Now reduction process is started. The first step of reduction is, to reduce the articular surface anatomically. The articular surface should be reduced in such a way that there should not be any gap at the fracture site. AO reduction clamps are used to hold the reduction along the medial and lateral condyles. If there is a gap or comminution between capitellum and trochlea process then the clamp should not be tightened too much to achieve compression. Instead the length of the articular surface maintained with graft in between. But when there is no bone loss then compression can be achieved by tightening the AO reduction clamp. Once the intercondylar compression is achieved then it is temporarily fixed with K wires. Attention is then diverted to the reduction of medal and lateral column over the intercondylar fracture fragments. Both the medial and the lateral columns are placed over the condylar fragments. Olecranon fossa serves as a guide for us and olecranon fossa congruity has to be maintained while reducing the fracture fragments. Once reduced this is temporarily fixed with K wires. Now once the temporary reduction is done we take over for the transosseous fixation of the intercondylar fragments. The transosseous fixation starts with a guide wire for 4 mm cannulated cancellous screw being passed from lateral condyle humerus to the medial condyle of the humerus such that it is very close to the joint surface about 1 cm above the joint surface.

The guide wire is directed posterolaterally to anteromedial direction and it is superiorly directed such that it doesn't cross the joint. By osteotomy approach one can see the guide wire coming out on the medial condyle and that it has not pierced the articular cartilage can be easily identified. Once the guide wire comes out on medial side it can be felt and seen and ulnar nerve should be protected medially. The guide wire should come out through the medial condyle. The position of the guide wire can be confirmed with the image intensifier and readjustments done if necessary under it. Once the position of the guide wire is confirmed, take another guide wire and pass it from lateral condyle 1 cm above the previous guide wire directed from the anterolateral aspect of the lateral condyle superiorly to the posteromedial aspect of the medial condyle. The two wires should be around 1 cm to 1.5 cm apart. If there is a difficulty in passing guide wire from the lateral condyle to medial condyle a wire can be passed from medial condyle to lateral condyle. Both the positions of the guide wire are checked under image intensifier whether it has pierced the joint or not. The first guide wire is drilled with a cannulated drill bit to create a tunnel of size 4 mm so that a cannulated screw of 4 mm can be passed from lateral to medial side of appropriate length. The length should be such that it engages both the medial and lateral condyles in reduced position. Then through a second guide wire a cannulated drill bit is passed to create a second tunnel of 4 mm above the first one. This tunnel is directed anterolateral to posteromedial direction. Keeping

37

cannulated drill bit in situ disconnect the drill. Take a straight stainless steel wire of 18 gauze, pretension it outside, and then pass the stainless steel wire through the cannulated screw so that it comes out on the medial side. Grab the wire from medial side. Bend it slightly and pass a small washer slightly bigger than the size of 4 mm. Turn that stainless steel wire and pass through the drill bit kept in situ from the medial aspect to the lateral aspect. Push the wire form medial to lateral aspect so that it comes out on the lateral side through the cannulated drill bit. Remove the cannulated drill bit now. Pull the wire tight so that the washer engages on to the mouth of the tunnel on the medial side. Remove the drill bit from the lateral side. Now take the wire tensioner and engage two ends of the wire onto it. Now start tensioning the stainless steel wire from the lateral side. As we tension the wires, we can both, feel and see the reduction occurring in the intercondylar region. The fracture site goes on compressing tightly and the stability of fracture goes on increasing, and a well felt rigidity is achieved. The rigidity, stability and the compression achieved as a result of this is such great that we feel satisfied and ensure that the intercondylar fracture is fixed quite well. The stability and strength of the fixation can be checked on the table by moving the joint freely in both anterior posterior and mediolateral direction. Over this the fixation of the two columns can be achieved by using two anatomical plates which can be comfortably placed over this. If the bone is osteoporotic and doesn't hole the implant well then a technique of multiple K wire along with stainless steel wires could be added over this tranosseous fixation or a transosseous transcolumnar cannulated screws along with tunnel can be done with the same transosseous technique could be achieved for the bicolumnar reconstruction.

The fixation achieved by this procedure is bicorticular, which cannot be achieved by any fixation device in low intraarticular fractures of lower end of humerus. The fixation achieved is very rigid, stable and bicortical. The stability achieved is such great that a very early mobilization is possible by using this technique. This technique also gives freehand for the application of the anatomical plate and its screws comfortably in the metaphyseal region.

Osteoporotic fracture fixation

In osteoporotic fractures the anatomical plates and reconstruction plates sometimes do not hold well. In these fractures the intercondylar element is fixed by transosseous technique, while the column fixation is done by K wires and stainless steel wire fixation. In this technique two K wires are passed from the medial and lateral condyle simultaneously so that they come out from the lateral and media supracondylar cortex respectively. The stainless steel wire is hooked along with the K wires which comes out laterally passed from the medial side to the K wire which is passed from the lateral condyle to the medial cortex. The tensioning of the stainless steel wire is done along the lateral column, similar procedure is done on the medial column also. This gives both the column fixation along with the intercondylar fixation of the fractures around elbow in osteoporotic patents.

The Column fixation

The column fixation can also be done by transosseous technique by the method described below

After fixing the intercondylar fracture the transosseous tension band wire technique, a guide wire is directed from lateral condyle of humerus upwards so that it crosses the supracondylar fracture complex and the wire comes out from the medial cortex of humerus. Similarly one more guide wire is passed about 1 cm to 2 cm above the first guide wire and in the same direction and almost parallel to previous guide wire. A 4 mm cannulated drill bit is applied to the drill and is drilled though the first guide wire so that is comes out medially. A 4mm cannulated screw of appropriate length is applied. Though the second guide wire cannulated drill bit of 4 mm is drilled creating a tunnel of 4mm above the previous tunnel. A stainless steel wire is passed through the cannulated screw and is take out from the medial side. A washer of size greater than 4 mm is passed through the stainless steel wire medially and the stainless steel wire is bent and passed through the tunnel having the cannulated drill bit situ from the medial to lateral side. Now as the cannulated drill bit is removed the two ends of the stainless steel wires can be seen on the lateral side. Now the tensioner is applied to both the ends of the stainless steel wire laterally.as the tension is applied the washer blocks the upper tunnel medially and we can see and feel the fracture getting compressed. After full tension a rigid and stable reconstruct is achieved. The same procedure is done for the medial column fixation. In this way by transosseous tension band wire technique we can fix both the columns and the intercondylar fractures.

Once the fixation of the columns and intercondylar fracture is done, the fixation of the olecranon osteotomy is performed. In this two K wires parallel to each other is passed from the olecranon into the ulnar and is fixed by stainless steel wires over these K wires by modified tension band wire technique. The suturing of the muscles to the medial and the lateral compartment is done. A drain is kept. The ulnar nerve if required is transported anteriorly. The facia and the subcutaneous tissue are sutured in layers and the skin is closed. A posterior POP slab is applied for one day for post-operative pain relief.

Intraop Images

After Exposure

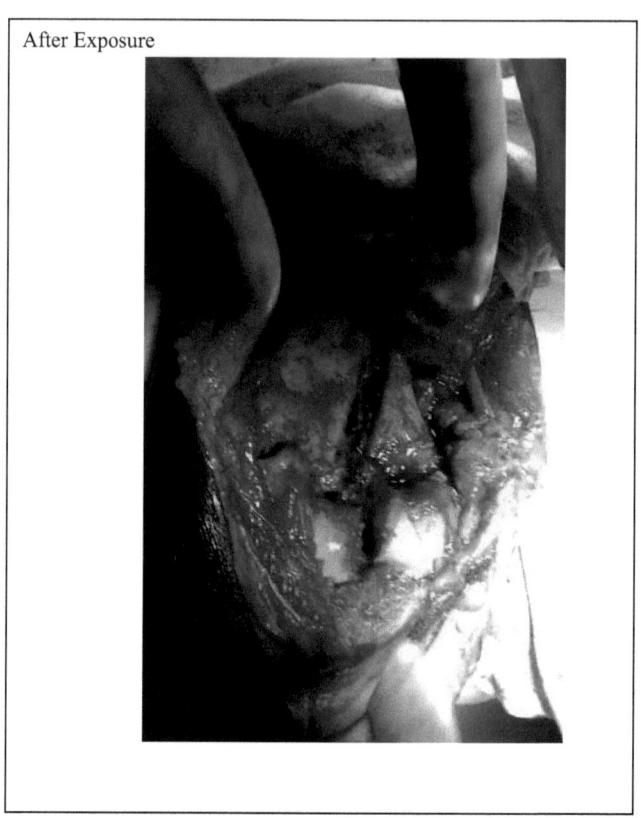

Holding intercondylar reduction with clamp

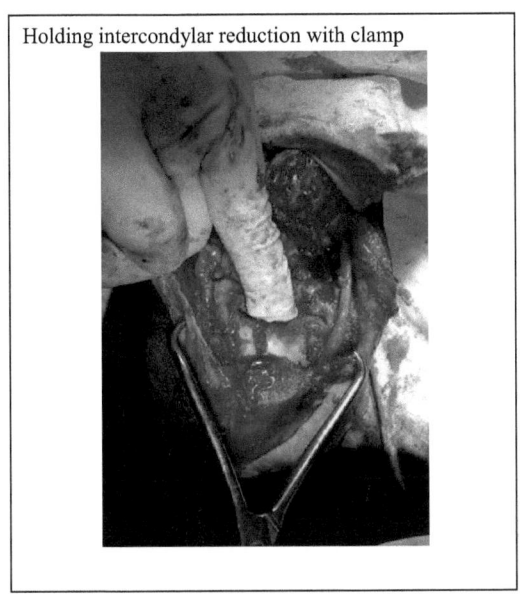

Passing guidewires in criss-cross fashion

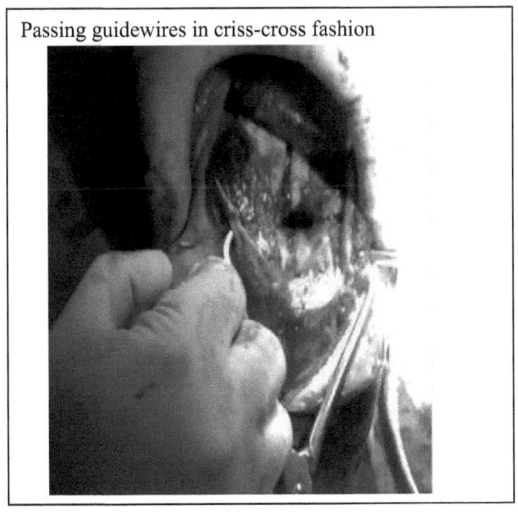

Drilling and insertion of one CC screw

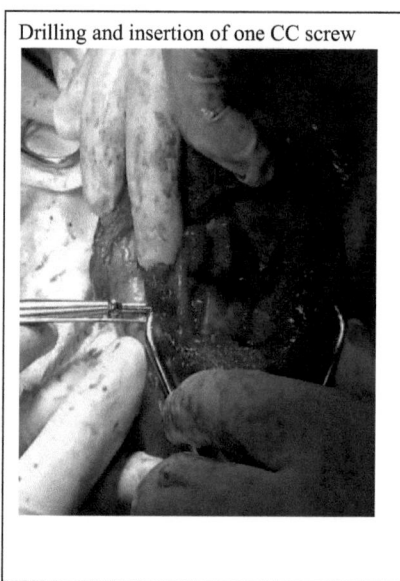

Insertion of stainless steel wire through cc
screw and cannulated drill bit over a washer

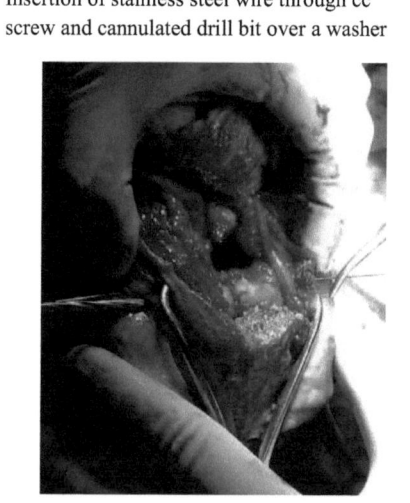

Final tightening of tension band wire over a screw and washer

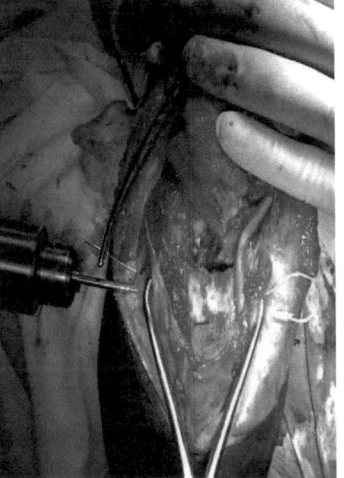

Final reduction for plating

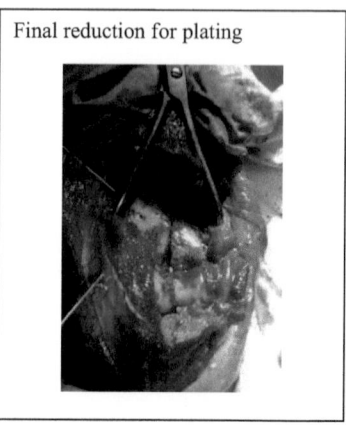

Intraop images over an image intensifier

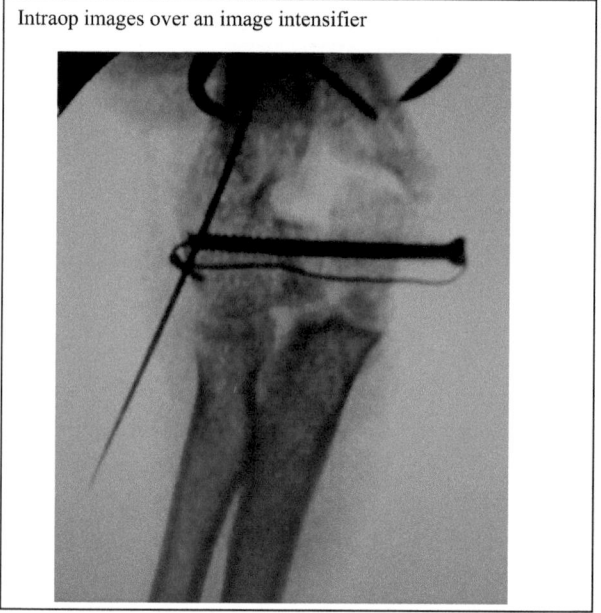

Pre op X-rays

AP   Lateral

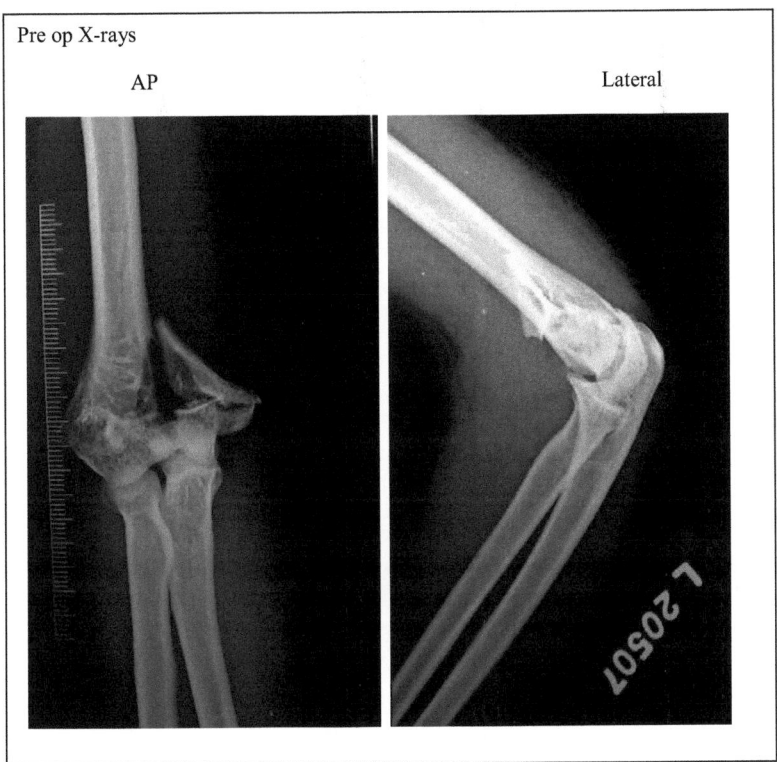

Post Op X-rays

AP   Lateral

TABLE 29-12 Surgical Pearls: "Checklist" for the Reconstruction of a Bicolumn Fractures

Admission checklist	Ensure no open wounds, skin tenting or areas of skin necrosis around the elbow
	Document any neurological deficit
	Ensure routine hematological, biochemical and cardiorespiratory work-up is performed
	Optimize any co-morbidities with medical treatment
	Explain risks of surgery to patient and likely prognosis
	Obtain informed consent
	Draw up a fracture plan based upon radiographs
	CT scan with 3D reconstruction for complex fractures
	Antithrombotic prophylaxis
	Heterotopic ossification prophylaxis in head-injured patients
Preoperatively	Discuss postoperative analgesia with anaesthetist (regional anesthesia if early postoperative passive movement is planned)
	Confirm availability of an assistant (preferrably "skilled")
	Antibiotic prophylaxis before tourniquet inflation
	Radiographer available for preoperative traction film and intraoperative radiographs
	Upper arm tourniquet
	Position patient—check supports
	Ensure free access to airway for the anesthetist before draping
	Drape iliac crest if bone grafting may be required
Equipment to be available in theater	Small and large fragment screw sets
	Small fragment plates and reconstruction plates
	Bending pliers and press for plate contouring
	K-wiring and tension band wire equipment
	Nerve slings
	Small oscillating saw
	Osteotomes
	Small and large reduction clamps
	Small cannulated screw set (if available)
	Hinged total elbow arthroplasty trays (if fracture may not be reconstructable)
Postoperatively	Liase with physiotherapist regarding rehabilitation protocol
	Update patient regarding surgical reconstruction obtained
	Wound check before discharge

APPLICATIONS OF OUR TECHNIQUE

We propose that our method of fixation can be widely used to fix fractures in the vicinity of the joint like the knee joint, ankle joint, wrist joint and shoulder joint.

- It can be used in fresh and old intercondylar fractures of humerus and femur.
- Unicondylar fractures of distal end humerus, distal end femur etc.
- In comminuted fractures where screw hold is not good, this technique, which gives four cortices fixation with good compression and can hold comminuted fragments as well.
- In fractures in osteoporotic bone were large implants can have shattering effect and screw may loosen out, this stainless steel compression gives good hold without fear of loosening and gives good hold without much implants.
- In non-union cases where good compression and rigid fixation is required which is definitely provided by this technique and the chances of healing would increase.
- In case of infected fracture as the implant used in very less and we can apply antibiotic beads along with it on both the sides. So that the infection is taken care of by the antibiotic beads and fixation is done by the stainless steel wire. We can avoid cannulated cancellous screws in infected cased and instead of screws only bony tunnels with stainless steel wires and washer would be the only implants used to fix.
- In open fractures our technique would be useful as a primary method of fixation as the hardware used is very minimal and compression, rigidity and stability achieved is of the highest level.
- In cases where there is complete bone loss e.g. loss of lateral condyle of humerus in osteoporotic fractures, our technique can be used along with illac crest along with facia over it as a graft to reconstruct the elbow joint.

Extended Applications:

This method can also be applied in following cases:

- Other intercondylar areas like upper end of tibia, femoral condylar area, distal radius etc.
- Unicondylar fractures of distal end humerus, femur or proximal tibia

In the fractures of proximal tibia, we can use our technique to fix the condyle rigidly and to get four cortices fixation. We can also get multiplaner fixation with our technique. Let us see in detail how it can be done. Firstly the condyles fixation with cannulated cancellous screw and a parallel

bony tunnel through which stainless steel wires are passed and it is tightened either on the media
l side or the lateral side. This fixation gives four cortices purchase and no loosening of the implant
and rigid fixation in both young patient and old osteoporotic patients.

Secondly for the fixation of posterio medial or posterio lateral fragment screws can be passed
from posterior to anterior direction through the posterio medial fragments and a parallel bon
tunnel is created along its side and then stainless steel wires are passed through the cannulated
screw and the bony tunnel and compression is achieved by tightening anteriorly. A good and
stable reconstruct is achieved by this technique.

We can cross the cannulated cancellous screw in the bone itself while fixing the condyles together
so that the bony tunnel and the cannulated screws they cross each other. So when the stainless
steel wire is passed through the cannulated screw and the bony tunnel, the stainless steel wire
would cross each other in the figure of eight, when compression is given in this way it will reflect a
transosseous tension band wiring being done. This is what we refer to as transosseous tension
band wiring.

DISCUSSION

Till date we have treated 10 patients of supracondylar fracture of humerus with intercondylar extension at in Shree Harilal Bhagwati Municipal General Hospital, Borivali (w), and Mumbai. In all 10 cases we got rigid and stable anatomical reduction on table itself which we confirmed by direct visualization under fluoroscopy. All patients were selected randomly the only criteria was a supracondylar fracture of lower end of humerus with intercondylar extension. We included all fresh fractures, non-union, compound fractures, and osteoporotic fractures. All patients were operated in prone position under region block or general anaesthesia. We used posterior approach of elbow with olecranon chevron osteotomy. Intercondylar portion of fracture was first reduced and held with AO reduction clamp as anatomical as possible. Then we passed a guide wire for cannulated cancellous screw from medial side to lateral aspect in intercondylar area crossing fracture perpendicularly. A second guide wire was passed through intercondylar area parallel to first one just distal to it without breaching the articular margin. A cannulated cancellous drill bit was used to drill the first guide wire from medial to lateral side. One proper size 4mm cannulated cancellous screw was passed over a guide wire and screw was placed in position. A cannulated drill bit was used to drill the second guide wire from lateral to medial side. Now the second guide wire was removed from drill bit. A pre-tensioned stainless steel wire was passed through the cannulated drill bit from lateral aspect to medial side. A medial end of same stainless steel wire now turned and passed through the medial side of cannulated screw head .so that it came out from the cannulated cancellous screw from lateral side. Now the cannulated cancellous drill bit was removed. Now the stainless steel wire is ultimately passing through transosseous canal into the lower intercondylar region and back again through cannulated cancellous screw in the upper part of the intercondylar region. Now tension was applied by twisting the two free ends of the stainless steel wire on the lateral side the intercondylar region. While tension was being applied we could feel the compression being achieved at the intercondylar region and also the rigidity was experienced as he tension was applied. This could be appreciated on fluoroscopy also. Added to these wires are passed from common extensor origin at lateral condyle and from common flexor origin at medial condyle. As both muscle group contracts, the distraction forces created by them are converted into compression forces by this Transosseous tension bend wiring. This method gave us four cortices fixation in the lower intercondylar region which was not possible till date by other methods of fixation. In osteoporotic fractures we used washer over the stainless steel wire to achieve compression at intercondylar region. In cases of non-union we did not used any graft in the intercondylar region, only freshening and compression was the modality of fixation. In cases of open fractures we constructed two transosseous canal instead of one and did not used cannulated cancellous screw as we intended to use very minimal implants. So now T-Y elbow type of fracture is converted into a supracondylar fracture. Rest fixation of supracondylar fracture was done with perpendicular plating and k wire TBW in case of osteoporotic bones. Out of 10 treated cases with this method all get rigid fixation and radiological union at average of 8 weeks. The maximum period for union was 12 weeks and the minimum time duration was 7 weeks. Average ROM was 5-100 with maximum range of motion (ROM) 0-110. One case had postoperative infection which was treated successfully by local debridement and antibiotics, one had k wire impinging on skin which was removed after radiological union and two patients lost follow up after 3 months.

Distal humerus fractures remain a challenging reconstructive problem for orthopaedic surgeons. Much of the difficulty encountered in treating distal humerus fractures lies in the complex anatomy of the elbow joint.[1] The highly constrained nature of the elbow joint causes it to absorb energy following direct trauma.[3] Consequently, articular comminution may occur. The distal humerus has a narrow supracondylar isthmus with a sparsity of adequate subchondral metaphyseal supporting bone, especially within the olecranon fossa.[4] The osteopenia observed in elderly patients adds to the complexity. Hastings and Engles have described a "spillover effect," in which inadequate restoration of a singularly injured joint can lead to abnormal wear and degenerative changes in an adjacent articulation. This effect can apply to the elbow [5-7]. However, Early mobilization , anatomical reduction and rigid fixation is required to prevent future problems.[8] We here described such one method which allow good compression at fracture site, rigid fixation and less hardware which is best for condylar area of elbow . Early mobilization is possible because of rigid fixation and good compression. In our method of intercondylar fixation rigid fixation and compression is achieved by transosseous route utilizing the principle of tension band wiring. Tension bend principle is applied here by the common extensor origin at lateral condyle and common flexor origin at medial condyle. As both muscle group contracts, the distraction forces created by them are converted into compression forces by this transosseous tension bend wiring. We hereby achieved four cortices fixation which is not described by any implant. Because of immense rigidity and stability we can mobilize the patient very early and the tension bend wiring technique acts in dynamic mode when muscles contracts. The added advantage of this modality is that it allows other implants for fixation of both supracondylar and intercondylar fracture over and does not interfere with instrumentation or implants. We propose that this method of fixation can have wide applications like: In fresh and old intercondylar fractures. In comminuted fractures were screw hold is not good, and this technique gives four

51

cortices fixation with good compression and can hold comminuted fragments as well. In fractures in osteoporotic bone were large implants can have shattering effect and screw may loose out, this stainless steel compression gives good hold without fear of loosening and gives good hold without much implants. In non-union cases were good compression and rigid fixation is required which is definitely provided by this technique and the chances of healing would increase. In case of infected fracture as the implant used in very less and we can apply antibiotic beads along with it on both sides, and we can do only Transosseous TBW without cannulated screw. This method can also be applied to other intercondylar areas like upper end of tibia, femoral condylar area, and distal radius. We can apply in more than one plane also like in upper end tibia it can be passed in medial to lateral plane and anterior to posterior direction, so we can take care of posterior fragment as well. Future technology may hold many solutions. With the advent of newer, stronger biocompatible materials, diverse hardware options allow improved reduction and fixation of distal humerus fractures. Lower profile plates and smaller screws are showing some results.

This method of transosseous intercondylar tension band wiring can be useful technique in such situations that allow the surge on to maintain the original articular congruity needed to prevent posttraumatic arthritis, which allows for faster and progressive postoperative rehabilitation.

Table-1: Management and follow up of patients							
Sr. No	Age	Sex	Mode of Injury	Management	Radiological Union	Functional Outcome (ROM*)	Complications
1	55 years	F	Fall from height	Interosseous TBW** + Perpendicular plating	10 weeks	0°-115°	K wire impingement on skin
2	38 years	M	Road traffic Accident	Interosseous TBW + Perpendicular plating	7 weeks	5°-115°	No major complications
3	65 years	F	Fall on Ground	Interosseous TBW + Perpendicular plating	10 weeks	5°-110°	No major complications
4	47 years	M	Road traffic Accident	Interosseous TBW + Perpendicular plating	9 weeks	10°-110°	No major complications
5	85 years	F	Fall on Ground	Interosseous TBW + K wire TBW for both columns	12 weeks	10°-95°	Superficial infection (lost follow up after 3 months)
6	46 Years	M	Road traffic accident	Interosseous TBW + Perpendicular plating	8 weeks	10°-100°	No major complications
7	53 Years	F	Road Traffic Accident	Interosseous TBW + Perpendicular plating	10 weeks	10°-95°	No major complications
8	28 Years	M	Road Traffic Accident	Interosseous TBW + Perpendicular plating	7 weeks	0°-115°	Lost follow up after 2.5 months (10 weeks)
9	42 years	M	Road Traffic Accident	Interosseous TBW + Perpendicular plating	8 weeks	5°-100°	No major complications
10	47 years	M	Road Traffic Accident	Interosseous TBW + Perpendicular plating	9 weeks	5°-110°	No major complications

* ROM = Range Of Motion; ** TBW = Tension Band Wiring; M= Male; F = Female

COMPLICATIONS

148. Hastings H, Graham TJ. The classification and treatment of heterotopic ossification about the elbow and forearm. Hand Clin 1994;10:417–437.

Wound Infection:

Often it is difficult to distinguish between a superficial infection, and mild wound hematoma or erythema, especially if cultures are equivocal. Broad-spectrum antibiotic therapy and topical dressings are often given empirically following discharge from hospital, and most superficial infections resolve on this regime. The risk of deep infection is higher with open fractures, particularly when there is gross contamination, or soft-tissue and bone loss.

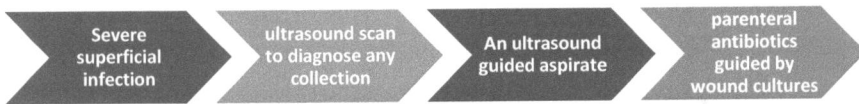

Severe superficial infection → ultrasound scan to diagnose any collection → An ultrasound guided aspirate → parenteral antibiotics guided by wound cultures

Early deep infection with stable internal fixation should be treated with a protocol of repeated surgical irrigation and debridement, and parenteral and topical antibiotic therapy. Subsequent non-union frequently occurs and requires bone grafting once the infection has been eradicated.

Deep infection may be refractory to this treatment protocol, and failure of the internal fixation usually occurs in these circumstances. In older patients, radical debridement, metalwork removal, and excision of the distal humerus may sometimes be effective in controlling infection, to allow later insertion of a hinged TER or arthrodesis.

In younger patients, salvage of the articular surface may be achieved after metalwork removal by the use of a fine-wire external fixator to provide skeletal stabilization, while infection is brought under control. Subsequent, internal fixation and bone grafting procedures have been successful in promoting aseptic healing in small numbers of patients with resistant infections.

Non-union/ Malunion and Fixation Failure.

Despite the advances in fixation techniques, fixation failure and non-union continue to occur, and pose their own set of challenges to reconstruction.

Definition and Classification

The terms fixation failure and non-union commonly occur at the level of the transcolumnar fracture. The fixation is typically used to refer to implant failure occurring at an early stage after surgery, whereas the latter is used to describe a more delayed failure of union. Non-union have been classified, using Weber and Cech guidelines, into hyper vascular (hypertrophic) and avascular (atrophic) types, whereas Mitsunaga classified non-union according to their anatomic locations.

Fixation failure appears as an implant breakage, migration, or loosening while non-union is easily detected by pain, loss of function, and abnormal movement at the fracture, at more than 6 months after the injury. Non-union in these circumstances usually presents with pain and x-ray-apparent widening of the fracture gaps, and/or delayed loosening or breakage of internal fixation. The risk of non-union using modern treatment methods is 6% (range 0% to 25%) with substantial number of bicolumnar fractures. Higher rates of non-union are being identified in patients with low osteoporotic fractures, improper and inadequate fixation of distal end humerus fractures.

Clinically patients present with pain, stiffness, and loss of function. Pain may be due to instability at fracture site, ulnar neuritis, or from posttraumatic osteoarthritis. If there is a failure, the elbow will frequently be unstable due to gross movement at the site of the fracture but it could be absent in case of fibrous union or implants in situ which is providing some degree of stability.

Treatment

It is important to establish the cause of failure of union. However, it is mandatory to exclude infection as a contributory factor to non-union before any further attempts at reconstruction, especially if the original fracture was open, or there was delayed wound healing after the original surgery. If fixation failure with separation of fragments is recognized at an early stage, immediate reoperation should be considered, especially if the original surgery was technically inadequate. Cast immobilization offers the best option at the beginning when the implant failure or loosening is suspected which offers time for union without further surgery. We prefer this option for the treatment in older patients with osteopenia to osteoporosis. Early revision can restore the stability, but there is a risk of introducing infection or further postoperative complications. However this option is preferred for younger individuals who need rigid fixation and early healing.

Non-union after non-operative treatment is difficult to treat owing to the complex mal-orientation of osteoporotic fracture fragments. We prefer to treat such fractures with rigid internal fixation and bone grafting. However, this is not without risks, and there may be particular technical problems encountered due to scarring from previous surgical approaches, broken implants, infection, gross osteopenia from previous fixation, and the viability of articular surface fragments. Revision to an arthroplasty is also the procedure of choice in elderly patients with limited functional expectations, and in patients with advanced arthritic change in their elbow.

Essential adjuvant treatment includes ulnar neurolysis and transposition, and radical soft-tissue release with capsulectomy to increase the arc of movement. With non-union surgery, anterior and posterior capsular releases, and ulnar nerve transposition are important adjunctive components of this procedure. Postoperatively, aggressive early mobilization of the elbow is important to retain the movement regained intraoperatively.

The risk of complications from revision ORIF is high and the functional outcome is frequently imperfect, not demonstrated significant deterioration in these results or progression to osteoarthritis of the joint. Total elbow arthroplasty, using a non-custom semi constrained hinge design, is used to treat unsalvageable non-unions.

If the patient has had a well-healed olecranon osteotomy following previous surgery, simple hardware removal is performed and either a triceps-reflecting or triceps-splitting approach can be used. If there is a non-union of an olecranon osteotomy, the elbow is approached through the non-union. This is then repaired with either tension band wiring or no absorbable sutures , after prosthetic insertion,

Other Techniques: Intramedullary nailing and Transcondylar rod techniques, osteochondral allograft replacement of the distal humerus, joint distraction, or interposition arthroplasty. Arthrodesis has a limited role to play in the treatment of the patient who has had multiple failed attempts at reconstruction, or in whom deep sepsis cannot be eradicated.

It is the author's policy to attempt revision internal fixation and bone grafting, combined with soft-tissue release and ulnar nerve decompression, wherever possible in younger individuals, aged 60 or under. This is because of concerns regarding the longevity of hinged TER in patients with prolonged life expectancy. The author reserves the use of TER for elderly symptomatic patients who are intolerant of an orthosis and for the rare instances in younger patients where excessive bone loss or osteoarthritis dictates that revision internal fixation is unlikely to produce a satisfactory outcome.

Malunion following bicolumnar fracture may occur either in the metaphysis of the distal humerus from mal-reduction of the transcolumnar fracture, or in the joint surface from mal-reduction of the articular fracture. It is likely that minor degrees of subclinical rotational deformity, procurvatum/recurvatum, and varus/valgus deformity commonly occur following the reconstruction of complex comminuted bicolumnar fractures.

Extensive procurvatum or recurvatum may cause loss of flexion or extension movement, whereas cubitus varus and valgus deformity may cause significant cosmetic deformity, instability, or may be associated with ulnar neuritis.

Nerve Injury

Neural injuries are commonly associated with bicolumnar fractures and are classified according to when they occur, the nerves involved, and the severity of the neural injury. Nerve injury may vary in severity from minor dysesthesia, to complete sensory loss and paralysis. Intraoperative nerve division, manipulation and devascularization, inadequate release, impingement, or injury by bony fragments or hardware, and postoperative fibrosis may all contribute to the development of neural problems after surgery. Ulnar neuritis may develop at a later stage of treatment, and may be associated either with non-union or a cubitus valgus deformity.

The ulnar nerve is the most commonly involved, both at the time of injury and intraoperative due to its close anatomic relationship with the medial epicondyle, and is particularly at risk if there is wide displacement of the columns. During ORIF, the ulnar nerve is more at risk in triceps-reflecting approaches, or if it is not transposed. The radial nerve is at risk with triceps-splitting approaches, if the split is continued too far proximally. More specialist evaluation of ulnar nerve palsy may be undertaken using the McGowan classification, the Gabel score, or the PRUNE score.

Nerve exploration is mandatory if dysfunction is detected prior to surgical intervention, particularly with penetrating trauma. If the nerve is found to be intact, it must be fully decompressed, whereas if the nerve is transected, an immediate repair is undertaken. It is important that decompression is performed at all possible levels of compression, including the arcade of Struthers (5 cm above the medial epicondyle), the medial intermuscular septum, the cubital tunnel, the flexor carpi ulnaris (Osborne) arcade, and the deep aponeurosis of the common flexor mass. A radial or median nerve palsy detected postoperatively requires early reexploration, as these nerves are not routinely identified and surgical injury must be excluded.

The prognosis for most nerve injuries in continuity is good, but the recovery is much more variable following transection or avulsion. This emphasizes the importance of adequate protection and anterior transposition of the ulnar nerve away from implanted hardware and bony fragments at time of the primary surgery.

Elbow Stiffness and Heterotopic Ossification

The elbow is prone to stiffness after trauma because of the high degree of congruency of the joint and the proximity of the brachialis anteriorly to the capsule, which forms scar tissue and heterotopic bone after injury. Furthermore the degree of stiffness often improves gradually with time. Most active individuals complain of functional disability and require treatment more for younger patients who are in manual work, or who are keen to return to playing sport.

In a large series of elbow contractures, it was estimated that one-third were due to fractures. Risk factors include severity of soft-tissue or bone injury, particularly of the articular surface, delayed surgery, advanced age, and prolonged immobilization after surgery.

Morrey has classified these into extrinsic, intrinsic, or mixed.

Stiffness type	Cause
Extrinsic	Heterotopic ossification and contractures of the anterior and posterior capsule, collateral ligaments, and muscles.
Intrinsic	Joint incongruity or osteoarthrosis: Intraarticular non-union or malunion of the fracture, osteophytes, loose fracture fragments, implant impingement (intra-articular screw placement, screws violating the olecranon fossa, and excessively low placement of column plates)
Mixed	Both extrinsic or intrinsic causes in combination

Heterotropic Ossification

The severity of postsurgical heterotopic ossification is variable and can be classified according to the system of Hastings. Prophylactic bisphosphonates, non-steroidal anti-inflammatory medication, or radiation may help to reduce the formation of heterotopic bone, but may retard bone healing.

TABLE 29-14 The Hastings[148] Classification of Heterotopic Ossification

Class	Subtype	Description
I		Radiographic heterotopic ossification without functional limitation
II	A	Limitation of flexion/extension
	B	Limitation of forearm pronation/supination
	C	Limitation in both planes
III		Bony ankylosis of either the elbow or forearm

Non-operative treatment should attempt to regain movement gradually, without precipitating inflammation. Oral non-steroidal anti-inflammatory medication and serial splinting may be useful in helping to regain movement, decreasing inflammation and pain. Closed manipulation under anaesthesia is not recommended due to the risk of iatrogenic fracture in comminuted, intercondylar unstable or osteoporotic fractures.

Radiologically, any heterotopic ossification must be corticated and quiescent. Open contracture release is most commonly performed, although arthroscopic capsular release is gaining in popularity. The surgery should be lesion-specific to address all components of the contracture

Lesion-specific surgery may include anterior and posterior capsulectomy for capsular contracture, subperiosteal elevation of the brachialis and triceps muscles, subtotal collateral ligament release and excision of all heterotopic bone. Postoperatively, adjuvant radiation, and medical therapy to prevent the re-formation of heterotopic bone have been recommended. It is important that movement is sustained in the early postoperative period, ideally using a continuous passive motion machine, with regional anaesthesia.

Osteoarthritis

Early rapid progression to symptomatic osteoarthrosis is due to inadequate restoration of articular congruity, early collapse of the articular surface despite a technically adequate ORIF or involve the whole articular surface , or occur segmentally, affecting either the trochlea or the lateral joint surface . Other causes of rapid post-surgical articular cartilage deterioration include loose bodies producing third-body wear and inadvertent intra-articular placement of metalwork. The radiological severity of osteoarthrosis may be classified using the scale of Knirk and Jupiter. Minor degrees of posttraumatic arthrosis are inevitable in later life following reconstruction of severe bicolumnar fractures in younger individuals.

The initial results of elbow replacement for osteoarthrosis were disappointing. However, satisfactory medium-term results have been reported more recently following refinements to prosthetic design, and restriction of the use of arthroplasty to older patients with low physical demands on their elbow. Total Elbow Replacement to Treat Acute Bicolumnar Fractures Currently the use of TER has been confined largely to elderly, low-demand patients with bicolumnar fractures that are not amenable to reconstruction by ORIF or who have pre-existing conditions of the elbow, most notably rheumatoid arthritis. Resurfacing arthroplasty may be used if both epicondyles are intact, and may be associated with lower rates of loosening, the use of a non-custom semi-constrained hinge is usually preferred, as it removes the risk of dislocation in patients with limited life expectancy.

The problem patient remains the younger active individual who develops early symptomatic posttraumatic osteoarthritis after a bicolumnar fracture. Currently the results of elbow replacements in these individuals are poor, with high rates of early loosening. The choice of treatment rests between non-operative treatment with orthotic and medical management, or non-prosthetic arthroplasty (either by resection, interposition, or distraction).

Instability

Instability is uncommon after these injuries because the collateral ligaments are intact and anatomic healing of the bicolumnar fracture will normally restore bony congruity. The elbow is therefore more at risk of stiffness from capsular scarring and fibrosis, than instability. If this is recognized early, a temporary external fixator, ideally of hinged design, should be used to augment the internal fixation for the first four weeks after surgery.

Olecranon Osteotomy Complications.

Prominence of the implants used to repair the olecranon osteotomy is common, and may lead to painful local symptoms or recurrent olecranon bursitis. Fixation failure, delayed union and non-union are not uncommon.

Some studies have suggested that this non-union of the osteotomy is more commonly associated with use of the tension band wiring technique, whereas others have shown higher rates with solitary screw techniques. Non-union and early fixation failure can be treated by revision internal fixation using a contoured ulnar plate, and bone grafting

CONCLUSION

Complicated fractures, open fractures, non-unions, metaphyseal fractures involving other joints and fractures of intercondylar region can be successfully managed by Transosseous tension band wire technique. We recommend such technique and welcome further research in this technique.

BIBLIOGRAPHY

1. Palvanen M, Kannus P, Niemi S, et al. Secular trends in the osteoporotic fractures of the distal humerus in elderly women. Eur J Epidemiol 1998;14:159â€"164.

2. Jupiter JB, Morrey BF. Fractures of the distal humerus in the adult. In: Morrey BF, ed. The elbow and its disorders, 2nd ed. Philadelphia: WB Saunders, 1993:328â€"366.

3. Rose SH, Melton LJ III, Morrey BF, et al. Epidemiologic features of humeral fractures. Clin Orthop 1982;24â€"30.

4. Robinson CM, Hill RM, Jacobs N, et al. Adult distal humeral metaphyseal fractures: epidemiology and results of treatment. J Orthop Trauma 2003;17:38â€"47.

5. Brannon JK, Woods C, Chandran RE, et al. Gunshot wounds to the elbow. Orthop Clin North Am 1995;26:75â€"84.

6. Zinman C, Norman D, Hamoud K, et al. External fixation for severe open fractures of the humerus caused by missiles. Ortho Trauma 1997;11:536â€"539.

7. Lerner A, Stahl S, Stein H. Hybrid external fixation in high-energy elbow fractures: a modular system with a promising future. J Trauma 2000;49:1017â€"1022.

8. Palvanen M, Niemi S, Parkkari J, et al. Osteoporotic fractures of the distal humerus in elderly women. Ann Intern Med 2003;139:Wâ€"W61.

9. Kannus P, Niemi S, Parkkari J, et al. Why is the age-standardized incidence of low-trauma fractures rising in many elderly populations? J Bone Miner Res 2002;17:1363â€"1367.

10. McKee MD, Jupiter JB. Fractures of the distal humerus. In: Browner B, Jupiter J, Levine A, et al, eds. Skeletal trauma, 3rd ed. Philadelphia, WB Saunders, 2003;1436â€"1480.

11. Amis AA, Miller JH. The mechanisms of elbow fractures: an investigation using impact tests in vitro. Injury 1995;26:163â€"168.

12. Kannus P, Parkkari J, et al. The injury mechanisms of osteoporotic upper extremity fractures among older adults: a controlled study of 287 consecutive patients and their 108 controls. Osteoporos Int 2000;11:822â€"831.

13. Campbell WC. Incision for exposure of the elbow joint. Am J Surg 1932;15:65â€"70.

14. Gschwend N, Loehr J, Ivosevic-Radovanovic D, et al. Semiconstrained elbow prostheses with special reference to the GSB III prosthesis. Clin Orthop 1988;104â€"111.

15. Gschwend N, Loehr J. [Elbow arthroplasty]. Orthopade 1980;9:158â€"168.

16. Olson SA, Hertel R, Jakob RP. The trans-tricipital approach for intra-articular fractures of the distal humerus: a report of two cases. Injury 1994;25:193–198.

17. Kasser JR, Richards K, Millis M. The triceps-dividing approach to open reduction of complex distal humeral fractures in adolescents: a Cybex evaluation of triceps function and motion. J Pediatr Orthop 1990;10:93–96.

18. McKee MD, Kim J, Kebaish K, et al. Functional outcome after open supracondylar fractures of the humerus. The effect of the surgical approach. J Bone Joint Surg Br 2000;82:646–651.

19. McKee MD, Wilson TL, Winston L, et al. Functional outcome following surgical treatment of intra-articular distal humeral fractures through a posterior approach. J Bone Joint Surg Am 2000;82-A:1701–1707.

20. Pajarinen J, Bjorkenheim JM. Operative treatment of type C intercondylar fractures of the distal humerus: results after a mean follow-up of 2 years in a series of 18 patients. J Shoulder Elbow Surg 2002;11:48–52.

21. Morrey BF, Bryan RS, Dobyns JH, et al. Total elbow arthroplasty. A five-year experience at the Mayo Clinic. J Bone Joint Surg Am 1981;63:1050–1063.

22. Bryan RS, Morrey BF. Extensive posterior exposure of the elbow: a triceps-sparing approach. Clin Orthop 1982;188–192.

23. Shahane SA, Stanley D. A posterior approach to the elbow joint. J Bone Joint Surg Br 1999;81:1020–1022.

24. Wolfe SW, Ranawat CS. The osteo-anconeus flap. An approach for total elbow arthroplasty. J Bone Joint Surg Am 1990;72:684–688.

25. Alonso-Llames M. Bilaterotricipital approach to the elbow. Acta Orthop Scand 1972;43:479–490.

26. Schildhauer TA, Nork SE, Mills WJ, et al. Extensor mechanism-sparing paratricipital posterior approach to the distal humerus. J Orthop Trauma 2003;17:374–378.

27. Morrey BF. Revision total elbow arthroplasty. In: Morey BF, ed. Joint replacement arthroplasty. New York: Churchill-Livingstone, 1991.

28. O'Driscoll SW. The triceps-reflecting anconeus pedicle (TRAP) approach for distal humeral fractures and non-union. Orthop Clin North Am 2000;31:91–101.

29. Kocher T. Textbook of operative surgery, 3rd ed. London: A and C Black, 1911.

30. Moran MC. Modified lateral approach to the distal humerus for internal fixation. Clin Orthop 1997;190–197.

31. Ring D, Jupiter JB, Gulotta L. Articular fractures of the distal part of the humerus. J Bone Joint Surg Am 2003;85-A:232â€"238.

32. Henry AK. Extensile exposure, 2nd ed. Baltimore: Williams & Wilkins, 1957.

33. Kelly RP, Griffin TW. Open reduction of T-condylar fractures of the humerus through an anterior approach. J Trauma 1969;9:901â€"914.

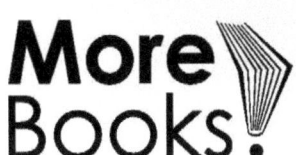
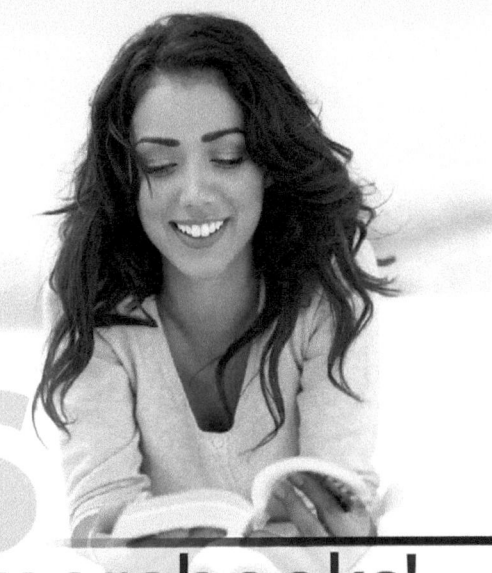
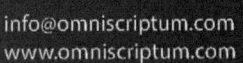
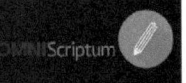

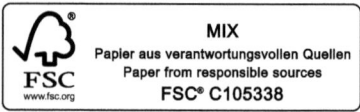
Printed by Books on Demand GmbH, Norderstedt / Germany